Class Struggle and Social Welfare

For too long the collective struggles of the oppressed over welfare provision and welfare settlements have been ignored, yet such struggles punctuate recent British history. By bringing together a series of case studies of episodes of collective action, *Class Struggle and Social Welfare* aims to rediscover this 'hidden history'.

In chronological format, the book presents some of the most important struggles in the development of welfare and social policy from the early nineteenth century through to the present day. Issues and topics covered include:

- the growth of capitalism
- the development of the Poor Laws and the anti-Poor Law movement
- working-class self-help welfare in the nineteenth century
- rent strikes on the Clyde in the 1920s
- the squatters' movement in the 1950s
- the struggle for abortion rights
- an analysis of the urban riots in the 1980s
- the great poll tax rebellion
- the growth of the mental health users' movement

Class Struggle and Social Welfare will be essential reading for those studying social policy, sociology, politics and history.

Michael Lavalette is a Lecturer in Social Policy at the University of Liverpool and **Gerry Mooney** is Staff Tutor in the Social Sciences with the Open University in Scotland.

The State of Welfare
Edited by Mary Langan

Throughout the Western world, welfare states are in transition. Changing social, economic and political circumstances have rendered obsolete the systems that emerged in the 1940s out of the experiences of depression, war and social conflict. New structures of welfare are now taking shape in response to the conditions of today: globalization and individuation, the demise of traditional allegiances and institutions, the rise of new forms of identity and solidarity.

In Britain, the New Labour government has linked the projects of implementing a new welfare settlement and forging a new moral purpose in society. Enforcing 'welfare to work', on the one hand, and tackling 'social exclusion' on the other, the government aims to rebalance the rights and duties of citizens and redefine the concept of equality.

The State of Welfare series provides a forum for the debate about the new shape of welfare into the millennium.

Titles of related interest also in *The State of Welfare* series:

Class Struggle and Social Welfare

Edited by
Michael Lavalette
and Gerry Mooney

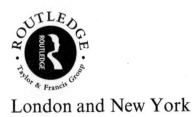

London and New York

First published 2000 by Routledge
11 New Fetter Lane, London EC4P 4EE

Simultaneously published in the USA and Canada
by Routledge
29 West 35th Street, New York, NY 10001

Routledge is an imprint of the Taylor & Francis Group

Typeset in Times by Taylor & Francis Books Ltd
Printed and bound in Great Britain by MPG Books Ltd,
Bodmin

British Library Cataloguing in Publication Data
A catalogue record for this book is available from the British
Library

Library of Congress Cataloging in Publication Data
Class struggle and social welfare/edited by Michael Lavalette
and Gerry Mooney
Includes bibliographical references and index
1. Public welfare–Great Britain–History. 2. Great Britain–
Social policy. I. Lavalette, Michael. II. Mooney, Gerry, 1960–.
III. Series.
HV245.C5984   2000
361.60941–dc21   99-052995

ISBN 0–415–20104–7 (hbk)
ISBN 0–415–20105–5 (pbk)

In memoriam: John Mooney (1920–1999)

Contents

Contributors

Michael Lavalette is a lecturer in Social Policy at the University of Liverpool. He writes on Marxism and social welfare, child labour and studies on protest action and collective struggle. His recent publications include a study of the Liverpool dock dispute, *Solidarity on the Waterfront* (LiverPress, 1997), and a history of child labour in Britain, *A Thing of the Past?* (Liverpool University Press, 1999). He is currently writing a book with Gerry Mooney and Iain Ferguson which takes a classical Marxist approach to social welfare (Sage, forthcoming). He is on the editorial board of the *International Socialism* Journal.

Gerry Mooney is staff tutor in the Faculty of Social Sciences at the Open University, Scotland. He is co-editor (with Steve Pile and Christopher Brook) of *Unruly Cities?* (Routledge, 1999). He is currently working with Michael Lavalette and Iain Ferguson on a book which reasserts the relevance of classical Marxism to the study of social welfare (Sage, forthcoming). He has also contributed chapters and articles to a number of volumes and journals in the fields of social policy and urban studies.

Mark O'Brien teaches in an East London Further Education College. He is the author of *Perish the Privileged Orders: A Socialist History of the Chartist Movement* (Redwords, 1995) and has also written against the influence of postmodernist theory in historiography in the collection *Essays on Historical Materialism* (J. Rees, ed., Bookmarks, 1998). He is on the editorial board of the *International Socialism* Journal.

Chris Jones is Professor of Social Policy and Social Work at the University of Liverpool. **Tony Novak** is a lecturer in Social Policy at the University of Liverpool. The authors – both individually and together – have researched and written on the history of social welfare in Britain and on its contemporary transformations, focusing respectively on social work and social security. They are the co-authors of *Poverty, Welfare and the Disciplinary State* (Routledge 1999) which charts the re-emergence of more punitive forms of social policy at the end of the twentieth century.

John Charlton taught History and Politics for thirty years at Leeds Polytechnic and at the University of Leeds. He has recently had two books published: *The Chartists: The First National Workers Movement* (Pluto, 1997) and *'It Just Went Like Tinder': The Rise and Fall of a Mass Movement* (Redwords, 1999). He is currently working on a study of the Great Unrest, 1910–1914. John Charlton is a long-standing member of the Socialist Workers Party.

Seán Damer teaches a course titled 'The sociology of modern Scotland' in the Department of Sociology at the University of Glasgow. He is the author of *From Moorepark to 'Wine Alley': The Rise and Fall of a Glasgow Housing Scheme* (Edinburgh University Press, 1989) and *Glasgow: Going For a Song* (Lawrence and Wishart 1990).

Alan Johnson is a Reader in Sociology and History at the Centre for Studies in the Social Sciences, Edge Hill College of Higher Education. He has written widely on the theme of collective action, including 'Militant and the failure of "acherontic" Marxism in Liverpool' (in C. Barker and P. Kennedy, eds, *To Make Another World*, Avebury, 1996), and is co-editor (with C. Barker and M. Lavalette) of two volumes on the collective struggle, *Constructing Strategies, Transforming Identities* (Liverpool University Press, forthcoming) and *Leadership and Social Movements* (Manchester University Press, forthcoming). He is currently working on a political biography of Hal Draper.

Laura Penketh and **Alan Pratt** are lecturers in Social Policy at the University of Central Lancashire. Both authors have written on aspects of political philosophy and social welfare, disadvantage and discrimination. Laura Penketh is completing a book on the Central Council for Education and Training in Social Work's anti-racist initiatives (Policy Press, forthcoming). Alan Pratt is co-editor of *Social Policy: A Conceptual and Theoretical Introduction* (Sage, 1997), and is presently working on a second edition of the text.

Charlie Johnstone is a lecturer in Sociology at the University of Paisley. He has published a number of articles on the subject of housing in

Glasgow. He is currently working on issues to do with housing and 'social exclusion'.

Sue Clegg is a principal lecturer in Social Research at Leeds Metropolitan University. **Rita Gough** was formerly employed at the University of Central Lancashire. She now works as a childcare specialist with Blackpool Social Services Department. They have both been researching the politics of abortion and the women's movement for several years and were active participants in many of the struggles to defend women's right to choose which are outlined in their chapter.

Rumy Hasan is a lecturer in the Business School at Leeds University. He researches and writes primarily on the social, political and economic problems of the emerging market economies of the former Soviet Union and Eastern Europe.

Iain Ferguson is a lecturer in Social Work in the Department of Applied Social Studies at the University of Paisley. His major fields of study are the mental health users' movement and Marxism and social work. He is currently working on a book with Michael Lavalette and Gerry Mooney which takes a classical Marxist approach to social welfare (Sage, forthcoming). Iain Ferguson is a long-standing member of the Socialist Workers Party.

Series editor's preface

State welfare policies reflect changing perceptions of key sources of social instability. In the first half of the twentieth century – from Bismarck to Beveridge – the welfare state emerged as a set of policies and institutions which were – in the main – a response to the 'problem of labour', the threat of class conflict. The major objective was to contain and integrate the labour movement. In the post-war decades, as this threat receded, the welfare state became consolidated as a major employer and provider of a wide range of services and benefits to every section of society. Indeed, it increasingly became the focus of blame for economic decline and was condemned for its inefficiency and ineffectiveness.

Since the end of the Cold War, the major fear of capitalist societies is no longer class conflict, but the socially disintegrative consequences of the system itself. Increasing fears and anxieties about social instability – including unemployment and homelessness, delinquency, drug abuse and crime, divorce, single parenthood and child abuse – reflect deep-seated apprehensions about the future of modern society.

The role of state social policy in the Clinton–Blair era is to restrain and regulate the destructive effects of market forces, symbolized by the Reagan–Thatcher years. On both sides of the Atlantic, governments have rejected the old polarities of left and right, the goals of both comprehensive state intervention and rampant free-market individualism. In its pursuit of a 'third way' the New Labour government, which came to power in Britain in May 1997, has sought to define a new role for government at a time when politics has largely retreated from its traditional concerns about the nature and direction of society.

What are the values of the third way? According to Tony Blair, the people of middle England 'distrust heavy ideology', but want 'security and stability'; they 'want to refashion the bonds of community life' and, 'although they believe in the market economy, they do not believe that the only values that matter are those of the market place' (*The Times*, 25 July 1998). The values of the third way reflect and shape a traditional and conservative response to the dynamic and unpredictable world of the late 1990s.

The view expressed by Michael Jacobs, a leading participant in the revived Fabian Society, that 'we live in a strongly individualized society which is falling apart' is widely shared (*The Third Way*, London: The Fabian Society, 1998). For him, 'the fundamental principle' of the third way is 'to balance the autonomous demands of the individual with the need for social cohesion or "community" '. A key New Labour concept that follows from this preoccupation with community is that of 'social exclusion'. Proclaimed the government's 'most important innovation' when it was announced in August 1997, the 'social exclusion unit' is at the heart of New Labour's flagship social policy initiative – the 'welfare to work' programme. The preoccupation with 'social exclusion' indicates a concern about tendencies towards fragmentation in society and a self-conscious commitment to policies which seek to integrate atomized individuals and thus to enhance social cohesion.

The popularity of the concept of social exclusion reflects a striking tendency to aggregate diverse issues so as to imply a common origin. The concept of social exclusion legitimizes the moralizing dynamic of New Labour. Initiatives such as 'welfare to work', targeting the young unemployed and single mothers, emphasize individual responsibility. Duties – to work, to save, to adopt a healthy lifestyle, to do homework, to 'parent' in the approved manner – are the common themes of New Labour social policy; obligations take precedence over rights.

Though the concept of social exclusion targets a smaller section of society than earlier categories such as 'the poor' or 'the underclass', it does so in a way which does imply a societal responsibility for the problems of fragmentation, as well as indicating a concern to draw people back – from truancy, sleeping rough, delinquency and drugs, etc. – into the mainstream of society. Yet New Labour's sympathy for the excluded only extends as far as the provision of voluntary work and training schemes, parenting classes and drug rehabilitation programmes. The socially excluded are no longer allowed to be the passive recipients of benefits; they are obliged to participate in their moral reintegration. Those who refuse to subject themselves to these apparently benign forms of regulation may soon find themselves the target of more coercive interventions.

There is a further dimension to the third way. The very novelty of New Labour initiatives necessitates the appointment of new personnel and the creation of new institutions to overcome the inertia of the established structures of central and local government. To emphasize the importance of its drugs policy, the government has created the new office of Drugs Commissioner – 'Tsar' – and prefers to implement the policy through a plethora of voluntary organizations, rather than through traditional channels. Health action zones, education action zones and employment action zones are the chosen vehicles for policy innovation in their respective areas. At higher levels of government, semi-detached special policy units, think-tanks and quangos play an increasingly important role.

The State of Welfare series aims to provide a critical assessment of social policy in the new millennium. We will consider the new and emerging 'third way' welfare policies and practices and the way these are shaped by wider social and economic changes. Globalization, the emergence of post-industrial society, the transformation of work, demographic shifts and changes in gender roles and family structures all have major consequences for patterns of welfare provision.

Social policy will also be affected by the demands of social movements – women, minority ethnic groups, disabled people – as well as groups concerned with sexuality or the environment. *The State of Welfare* series will examine these influences when analysing welfare practices in the first decade of the new millennium.

Mary Langan
February 1999

Acknowledgements

This book would not have been completed without the help and support freely given by a number of people. First, we would like to thank the contributors, each of whom met our strict deadlines and displayed an immense amount of patience as the laborious editorial tasks were undertaken. Second, we would like to thank the series editor, Mary Langan, for her support for the project, and our contact at Routledge, Fiona Bailey, who has been very helpful both with advice and when dealing with our queries.

A reader of the book at an early stage of preparation said they liked the proposal, that its themes had not been addressed for some considerable time (if at all), but wasn't it all a bit 'SWPish'. Why this should matter confuses us: books are rarely dismissed because their political conclusions are 'Labourist' or because the authors share a social-democratic or a conservative world view. But we suppose we have to respond. Several of the contributors to the volume (including ourselves) are members of the Socialist Workers Party in Britain, but, to paraphrase the House Committee on UnAmerican Activities, several of the writers 'are not now, nor have they ever been' members of the organization. This is not an SWP book; the chapters do not present any 'party line', indeed there is a fair degree of disagreement between many of the authors over some of the specifics of their argument or their general political conclusions. What unites the contributors is a commitment to re-emphasizing the relevance of class and the class struggle within analyses of social welfare developments.

The demands of completing a collection such as this eat into the various other activities you would like to take part in. In particular, we both have young families and would like to thank our partners and children for their patience as the book was being completed.

Finally, while this book was nearing completion John Mooney, Gerry's father, died suddenly. As someone who was committed to social justice and to the working-class struggle, he would have been in agreement with the political thrust of this book. We dedicate the book to his memory.

1 Introduction

Class struggle and social policy

Michael Lavalette and
Gerry Mooney

Introduction

In recent years there has been a notable shift in attitude with regard to Marx within academic and intellectual circles. In 1997 and 1998 several 'quality' newspapers in Britain ran feature articles on Marx, with J. Cassidy in the *Independent on Sunday* (7 November 1997) suggesting that he was the 'next big thinker'. Derrida, for so long *the* postmodern French intellectual, has suggested that Marx's 'inheritance was ... absolute and thoroughly determinate' (1994: 14). Balibar, who along with Althusser was one of the key proponents of a dehuman-ized, structural Marxism in the 1970s, has suggested that there is a need to reappraise the 'Hegelian Marxist' tradition (see Rees 1998). Meanwhile, the *Socialist Register* devoted its 1998 edition to a discussion of the Communist Manifesto and its relevance in the 1990s. The reasons for the 'return of Marx' are varied, but war and the preparation for war (for example in the Middle East, the Balkans, Somalia and Rwanda), economic crisis (especially in the Asian Tiger economies), the realization in the former Stalinist states of Eastern Europe of what marketization has meant for the living conditions of the vast majority of the population, and the return of mass movements and revolution (for example in Indonesia, South Korea, France and Germany) have all played a part in the re-evaluation of Marxist ideology.

A second, equally important, reason for a 'return to Marx' has been a growing disillusionment with the rampant relativism of postmodern theorizing. With regard to social policy and welfare writing, postmod-ern theory never obtained the dominant position which it managed to achieve in various other academic disciplines. But nevertheless, even social policy writers sympathetic to some 'postmodern concerns' now suggest that there is a need to 'pull back' from the edge. Fiona Williams, for example, has argued that there is a need to break 'the pure relativist impasse which some postmodernist thinking has reached and ... perhaps touch some dogged materialist universalism of class-centric theory' (1996: 61).

But while social class is (once again) recognized as an important social division within modern societies and contemporary social policy, it tends to be regarded either as a descriptor of influences on social policy (via political parties and/or trade unions) or it is interpreted as one of many social divisions which policies will impact upon; one of a range of co-equal oppressions (Thompson 1998). In this sense it is viewed in relation to policy outcomes. However, the notion that social class, as a 'collective agency', may have a role in shaping and/or resisting policy developments is marginalized in the literature.

Agency and social policy construction

As presently formulated, much social policy theorizing tends to portray social and welfare policy developments primarily as the outcome of one of a number of 'agents'. First are the accounts which focus on the role of the state bureaucracy and civil servants (Heclo 1974; Fraser 1984). Within this social policy tradition, key individuals are identified, for example, Chadwick and Beveridge, and accorded a central role in the development of social policy. Through identifying such 'great men', welfare policy is portrayed as a progressive and expansive instrument for taming the excesses of the free market, developing inclusionary citizenship rights and dealing with specific social problems 'for the benefit of society as a whole'. This tradition has been particularly powerful in histories of social and welfare policies and practices which are dominated by 'Whig' interpretations of developments (see Jones 1991; Fraser 1984). It would be facile to argue that civil servants or the state bureaucracy do not have a role in the forming and implementation of policies, but such perspectives fail to acknowledge the complexities surrounding welfarism and welfare expansion, the conflicts welfare settlements reflect and generate, both between and within classes, and the ideological assumptions which underpin welfare practices, for example, assumptions of gender and nation (see Williams 1989; Hughes and Lewis 1998; Lewis 1998).

A second type of approach emphasizes the role played by political actors in policy developments. This 'political model' includes a focus on the part played by 'important' individuals but more significantly centres on political parties and their ideological commitments to particular forms or modes of welfare system and delivery. In everyday discourse this is often depicted as the most important factor shaping welfare regimes. It is often assumed, for example, that in British social policy the Labour Party, or at least the Labour Party prior to its remake under John Smith and Tony Blair, provides a greater commitment to an inclusive and expansionist welfare state than that which has characterized previous Conservative governments, especially since 1979. Ironically, given the dominant hold of this perspective at the level of the 'political common sense', there is not a vast literature covering these themes, but Sullivan (1992), Hill (1993), and Ludlam and Smith (1996) reflect this general approach that politics is paramount.

Clearly there are certain strengths to this approach and it is important that we acknowledge some of these here. It is surely correct to focus on the role of the 1945 Labour government in shaping the Beveridgean welfare state, although any focus on the uniqueness of post-1945 events in Britain can lead to an underestimation of the significant degree of continuity between reforms during this period and Liberal welfare policies introduced earlier in the twentieth century. It can also lead to a neglect of the degree to which the post-war settlement, the so-called 'social democratic consensus' over welfarism was shared across the political spectrum in the 1940s and 1950s. Similarly, Ludlam and Smith (1996) are also right to stress the 'Thatcherization' of the Labour Party and its consequences for welfare in the late 1990s (see also Driver and Martell 1998; Jones and MacGregor 1998; Lister 1998).

Yet despite its merits, this approach also fails to take full account of the socio-economic context within which welfare developments occur. That is to say, a focus on the specifics of British welfare policies can fail to adequately explain why similar policy innovations took place in other European societies, both in the post-1945 period and from the early 1980s onwards, despite having political parties in power with commitments apparently at odds with such developments. Thus, for example, right-wing political parties presided over welfare expansion after the Second World War, and since the 1980s socialist governments in Spain, France and Sweden have been involved in bouts of welfare 'restructuring' which demonstrate strong similarities with the policies of the Conservative government under Margaret Thatcher in Britain.

An attempt to move beyond the limits of the 'pure' politics model is offered by Esping-Anderson (1990) and his construction of welfare regimes. His approach focuses on different forms of welfare settlements and attempts to explain these by reference to political and cultural traditions. In the most pervasive regimes (such as in Scandinavia), extensive welfare provision and coverage, and the decommodification of welfare, is a consequence of political settlements between different classes and important pressure groups. Central to this perspective is the 'labour mobilization thesis', an emphasis on the ability of socialist or labourist organizations to mobilize cross-class support for decommodified welfare. This model has the potential to be much more dynamic than the first two approaches, but Esping-Anderson's discussion of labour mobilization essentially refers to the mobilization of the labour and trade union bureaucracies. There is little exploration in his work of the role of wider class or collective actions around welfare issues and the effect that this has on welfare settlements.

There is a fourth type of approach which is characterized by various Marxist models of welfarism. Given the centrality of class conflict and class struggle to Marxist social theory one might expect the major pieces of social welfare writing in this tradition to include a substantial account and examination of the role of class struggle in shaping welfare and social policies. Certainly some of these themes have been present in the writings of British Marxist historians like John Saville (1983). Saville clearly suggests that collective action is an important factor that needs to be incorporated into an analysis of welfare developments. But in the major Marxist-inspired accounts of social welfare, class, as a collective agency of social change, is once again missing. James O'Connor (1973) for example, in a widely read and much cited account of the crisis of welfare states in the 1970s, is predominantly concerned with political and economic processes, fiscal crises and issues of legitimation. Similarly, Offe (1984) concentrates on issues of legitimation in advanced capitalist societies. Other Marxist theorists, such as Ian Gough (1979), do acknowledge that 'class struggle' is a key feature of late twentieth-century societies, but they fail to explore its specific relevance to social policy.

It is left to Norman Ginsburg in his 1979 work, *Class, Capital and Social Policy*, to argue that class struggle provides a context within which social policies must be assessed, although he appears to abandon this way of thinking in his subsequent work, *Divisions of Welfare* (1992), where class is used much more as a descriptive device to aid the understanding of socially divided societies.

In sum, then, the focus of many existing Marxist accounts of social welfare has been on the structural inequalities that exist within modern capitalist societies, the role of social welfare in promoting or sustaining ideological hegemony and social control and the functional benefits welfare developments may bring to modern societies. Of course it is right that such concerns should be central (see Lavalette 1997) but left at this point these analyses become too one-sided. Welfare also provides a collectively consumed social wage. As Gough notes: 'The welfare state exhibits positive and negative features within a contradictory unity' (1979: 11). Precisely because 'welfare' provision under capitalism is contradictory, in that it can contain at one and the same time elements of both social wage and social control, it is possible to comprehend why class mobilizations develop to demand welfare, to resist cuts in provision or to fight particular forms of welfare delivery or their covert or not so-covert assumptions about working-class lives and modes of living.

Although downplaying the role of class struggle in his later works, Ginsburg remains one of the few recent theorists in social policy in Britain to recognize that class should occupy centre stage in social policy:

> There remains a huge antipathy to using and operationalising the concept of 'class' in policy analysis, presumably for fear of its Marxist connotations. Yet ... class ... is manifestly fundamental to the social structure and therefore to analysing the functioning and impact of the welfare state.
>
> (Ginsburg 1992: 189)

The consequence of not focusing on collective class mobilizations around welfare issues has been to leave the field of 'welfare struggles' to a broadly postmodern politics and analysis structured around the concept of 'new social movements' or 'new social welfare movements'. Such a politics is based on two overarching premises. First, class and class conflict are both dated and narrow concepts. *Dated* because it is assumed that the working class is in decline (and thus easily sits with trite Blairite claims that we are all middle class now), and *narrow* because it is assumed that class only ever referred to male, skilled manual workers. Second, only that particular group of the oppressed can fight their oppression. Within such trends a politics of identity is dominant and the welfare demands are increasingly structured around notions of particularism rather than a universal politics of welfare need. These arguments are more fully considered in a recent paper by Ferguson and Lavalette (1999), but let's briefly address each in turn.

The end of the working class?

During the 1980s in Britain, claims that we were witnessing the 'end of the working class' acquired some prominence. But in essence, we would suggest, proponents of this thesis confuse the 'restructuring' of the working class, which is a process as old as capitalism itself, with the end of the working class. Thus, while it is true that the old industrial working class is smaller now than it was twenty years ago, it is no less true that whole sections of workers, including, for example, teachers, lecturers, and a range of welfare workers, now consider themselves part of the white-collar working class in a way that would have been inconceivable thirty years ago. In addition, and rather ironically, this thesis is extremely Eurocentric, for while the manual working class may have shrunk within the old industrial heartlands of capitalism, on a world scale the industrial working class has grown immeasurably (see Callinicos and Harman 1987).

Second, the above should emphasize that the working class is a far from narrow grouping. For Marxists, class is essentially a relationship between groups of people who have identifiable positions within the entire system of social production (de Ste Croix 1981). Class is objectively defined. Under capitalism the key determinant is whether one owns and/or controls the means of production or whether one is forced to sell one's labour power in order to survive. This requirement and relationship applies to people in a range of occupational locations (factories, mines, offices, shops and throughout the service sector) and those who, for whatever reason, either in the short or long term are unable to enter the labour market – the non-labouring working class (the sick, the unemployed, the elderly, those with 'caring' responsibilities, and so on). This latter group does not have discrete interests from those members of the working class in employment. For both sections their interests are best served by the destruction of the dominant system and organization of production which breeds their oppression and exploitation. For Marxists, the definition of the working class includes the vast majority of the population within modern societies – men and women, gay and straight, black and white, young and old, able-bodied and disabled. Whether they perceive themselves to be part of the working class is, at this level, immaterial. Class identification is much more likely to be forged in the conflicts which capitalism generates, in the repeated waves of protest that punctuate history, and it should not surprise us that when the waves recede, or in periods of low levels of class conflict, such identification is weaker (though it rarely disappears).

Marxism, class and oppression

The second theme of postmodern/new social welfare movement analysis rests on a politics of identity and oppression. Some of these themes are specifically dealt with in this book (especially chapters 6 and 12). But here we wish to outline the Marxist approach to fighting oppression. In modern societies the working class remains oppressed. As Smith notes:

> Even in the richest societies in the world ... the working class still experiences oppression. Oppression takes many forms: regressive taxation policies; inferior schools; substandard or inaccessible medical care; the prevailing ideologies ... even the siting of toxic waste dumps, never installed anywhere but in working class areas – the list goes on. Oppression is ... a product of a system based upon the rule of a tiny minority at the expense of the vast majority ... oppression is endemic to capitalism.
>
> (Smith 1994: 40)

Of course, there are also a range of other oppressions in society, for example those which are based on gender, race or sexuality, but these do not cut across class divisions. The middle-class businesswoman may be oppressed but she can also benefit from the oppression of women if, for example, she hires a child-minder or nanny on poverty wages (German 1989). During the riots in Los Angeles in 1992, both the Chief of Police and the Mayor of LA were black and both had undoubtedly suffered racism during their careers, but it is unclear what exactly they had in common with the black rioters from the central LA district (Davis 1993a and 1993b). It is in this sense that the notion of an equivalence of oppressions is unhelpful. It ignores the fundamental class divide within society and leads to what Callinicos has termed 'oppression-trumping': 'a process of differentiation *ad finitum* as various groups ... claim ... the special, and often specially acute, character of *their* oppression' (1995: 198).

The notion of a range of discrete and equivalent oppressions tends to lead to a pluralistic view of the world and oppressions, where we all, in one way or another, use our 'power' to oppress each other. The real power within capitalist societies, that of capital, becomes no more severe or 'abusive' than that of white working-class men in their social relationships with working-class women or black people, for example.

Further, within such prognoses, the class nature of the state is lost. The state becomes viewed increasingly as an arbiter operating between competing interests and a politics of 'particularism' is advocated where the oppressed will become involved in setting their own agendas and obtaining appropriate outcomes from a (benevolent?) state (Williams 1992). However 'radical' such pluralisms may claim to be, the reality is often to ignore, mirror or even reinforce, the unequal distribution of power within capitalism.

Such accounts of the world are also deeply pessimistic as oppression becomes eternal. Women's oppression, for example, becomes an inevitable, transhistorical category, part of the 'human condition', rather than a changing experience that has altered historically through each mode of production. For Marxists, oppressions must be related to the concrete experiences of social life within the capitalist mode of production. This does not mean that women's oppression, racism, gay oppression, etc., are simply reducible to the functioning or needs of the capitalist economy but that they occur and/or take their present form in ways that are mediated by the wider, complex social totality of modern capitalism (Rees 1998). It is this perspective which entails the possibility of a world free from oppression. If oppression is a feature of class societies then the *possibility exists* for a future free from oppression and exploitation, the question is, how do we achieve this?

This leads to a more fundamental reason, within the Marxist tradition (at least in its 'classical' form, Anderson 1976), for opposing *all* forms of oppression. It follows directly from Marx's view of the working class as not simply a *suffering* class but rather, by virtue of its position within the process of capital accumulation, as the *agent*, or potential agent, of a socialist transformation of society, as the 'gravedigger of capitalism'. Here, anything which divides workers and undermines their collective organization by persuading them to see other groups of workers as 'the enemy', be it women, blacks or gays, weakens the working class and prolongs and strengthens the domination of the ruling class. On the one hand, racism, sexism or heterosexism can give the white/male/straight worker a sense of belonging to the dominant group, despite feeling powerless and alienated in every other aspect of his existence. On the other hand, in times of crisis, it can provide a ready-made scapegoat, in the shape of the oppressed group.

Thus the politics of Marxism is one that fights all forms of oppression and exploitation and in the process argues a position of unity – of collective interest in the removal of capitalism. In this struggle the oppressed must 'free themselves' in two linked senses: first, free themselves from what Marx termed the 'shit of ages', any vestiges of racism, sexism, homophobia, etc., and second, that this must be part of the process of the self-emancipation of the working class – ordinary people using their structural capacities to create and reshape the social world.

Our case, therefore, is that within the hidden history of working-class welfare struggles we can witness, in embryo, the unifying themes of a universalist politics of human need, which contrasts sharply with the concerns of particularism, difference and disunity which the dominant postmodern politics treats as a virtue.

The structure of this book

The central task of this volume is to focus on class movements and struggles around issues of social policy and social welfare and, in so doing, to argue that social policy analyses need to acknowledge 'class struggle' as a *potential* factor shaping and constraining policy outcomes and collective responses to welfare and social policy. This is not to assert that class struggles mechanically or automatically lead to welfare and social policies being developed in particular ways at particular periods but to argue that class provides the context within which policies are developed, welfare states reorganized and in which groups get access or are denied access to welfare.

This book is organized in the following way. Chapters 2, 3 and 4 consider the context of capitalist development and class struggle within which social policies developed. In the chapters by Mark O'Brien and John Charlton, the broad debate and approach is outlined with a focus on poverty and the development of the Poor Laws (Chapter 2, O'Brien) and the links between class conflict and the growth of the interventionist state in the late nineteenth and early twentieth centuries (Chapter 4, Charlton). Sandwiched between these chapters, Chris Jones and Tony Novak remind us that in the nineteenth century working-class suspicion of, and hostility to, the state produced a tradition of self-help welfare steeped in notions of collectivism and solidarity.

In the remaining chapters, we focus on a series of what Klandermans (1997) has called 'episodes of collective action' around specific welfare struggles. Chapters 5 to 12 follow a broadly chronological order and have been chosen to emphasize the range of conflicts welfare struggles generate. In his chapter on the Clyde rent war, Seán Damer focuses on housing struggles in Clydebank in the 1920s. Following the success of the mass Glasgow Rent Strike of 1915 which secured state rent controls, and subsequently state housing in the Housing and Town Planning Act 1919, Damer highlights the continuing role of working-class mobilization in defence of rent controls against landlords, detailing the degree of organization and consciousness which existed. As Damer rightly notes, this was not simply a defensive protest. Through what were at times diverse struggles over housing conditions and the costs of housing, working-class people in places like Clydebank and beyond were able to challenge prevailing ideologies about housing for the working classes, and in so doing came in direct conflict with both the landlord class and other 'vested interests'.

In Chapter 6, Alan Johnson looks at the struggle of the Poplar councillors between 1919 and 1925. This episode is relatively well known but Johnson explores the events to offer a critical analysis of Fox-Piven and Cloward's seminal text, *Poor People's Movements: Why They Succeed How They Fail*. He argues convincingly that leadership, organization and strategy are central concepts for understanding the dynamism of collective action and that within such democratic mobilizations we can start to witness a progressive, transitional politics of human need to counterpose present concerns with particularism.

In Chapter 7, Laura Penketh and Alan Pratt look at the political response to mass unemployment in the 1920s and 1930s. Again the struggles of the unemployed in this period are well known, but Penketh and Pratt use this episode to explore what Hal Draper calls the 'two souls of socialism', the response of the Labour Party bureaucracy in opposition and government and that of the National Unemployed Workers Movement.

Chapter 8 brings us back to housing in Clydeside, this time focusing on the struggles over state housing provision in Glasgow during the 1950s. Throughout the twentieth century Clydeside has been synonymous with housing problems and conflict over housing provision. But while Charlie Johnstone and Seán Damer both look at issues on Clydeside, albeit during different time periods and in different contexts, protest over state housing provision has been a feature of other towns and cities across Britain. Johnstone again draws our attention to the centrality of housing issues in the mobilization of Glasgow's working class in the immediate post-war period. He makes it clear that working-class struggles for state provision of housing at the local level were instrumental in securing national level state housing legislation and winning legitimacy for the role of the state in control of housing costs and the provision of housing for the working class.

In their chapter on the struggle for abortion rights, Sue Clegg and Rita Gough provide a comparative analysis between Britain and the United States since the 1960s. Importantly, this chapter highlights the role that non-class-based reforming pressure groups can have in shaping policy. However, in drawing out key differences in the experiences of those involved in the campaigns in Britain and the US, Clegg and Gough highlight the way in which the campaigns in defence of abortion rights were embedded within the wider working-class and trade union movement in Britain, something which was notable by its absence in the US to the cost, they argue, of the pro-choice movement in that country.

Rumy Hasan's discussion of riots and urban unrest in Britain in the 1980s and 1990s is somewhat different from the other case studies in this volume in that he engages first and foremost with the dominant explanations of and approaches to the riots. Much has been written about these episodes of urban unrest and Hussan critically discusses the dominant perspectives. In particular he notes the role of mainly unemployed and unorganized working-class people, both black and white, in challenging state racism and hostile policing, in a wider context of declining job opportunities and deteriorating housing. The riots were, he claims, a generalized response to the large-scale abandonment of working-class communities by the state, with the exception of policing, and by major sections of private capital.

In Chapter 11, we look at the massive anti-poll tax movement of the late 1980s and early 1990s. We start by developing a political economy of the poll tax which emphasizes that the tax was a central piece of government legislation aimed at redistributing tax from the poor to the rich to increase inequality and force local authorities to privatize and cut local welfare services. In the face of this blatant attack on their standard of living and local welfare provision the anti-poll tax movement grew to involve almost 17 million people in a campaign of mass non-payment and mobilized substantial numbers on demonstrations outside council chambers and in the heart of the City of London. The movement not only defeated the tax, but it was also central to removing Margaret Thatcher as Prime Minister.

Finally, in Chapter 12, Iain Ferguson focuses on the mental health users' movement in the 1990s. Rejecting claims from a number of social policy academics that such a movement is representative of a 'new social movement' and using material from his own studies on such movements in Scotland, Ferguson shows that from being predominantly the 'objects' of state policies, the growth of the mental health users' movement has begun to challenge welfare and social practices and in so doing has begun to shape and influence the development of policies. Alliances with trade unions and other protest groups in defence of welfare services, in the face of government cutbacks, illustrates the potential for this movement to become a more effective campaigning force. Ferguson engages directly with debates over identity politics and argues that they are incapable of providing a basis for challenging the stigma and material inequality experienced by the vast majority of people with mental health problems and that class-based politics provide the only firm basis for such a challenge.

To conclude, these chapters represent a series of rich ethnographic studies of working-class collective struggles to do with welfare. The chapters are unified around the themes of working-class self-activity and organization from below. A number of the studies highlight competing strategies and different forms of protest and organization. Taken as a whole, they rescue, from those who would have them consigned to history simply as unique or one-off events, the important – *and continuing* – role of working-class protest in the development and delivery of welfare policy and practice. While such struggles did not – and do not – always lead to particular policy developments, they do create and recreate the wider political context within which social and welfare policies are implemented. Viewed from this perspective, class struggle and class as an agency of change is integral to our understanding of the development of social welfare.

2 Class struggle and the English Poor Laws

Mark O'Brien

Introduction

Rhetoric and policies on the question of relief to the poor by all western European governments over the last decade have reflected an underlying philosophy which we can recognize from much earlier epochs. Notions such as the 'deserving' and the 'undeserving' poor, the stigmatizing of poverty, the criminalizing of vagrancy and restrictions on the mobility of the poor are a largely continuous theme in the Poor Laws of the past as well as the present. Of course, in each era the precise application of such ideas and the social policies emerging from them are different and are adapted to the 'needs' of the time. The sense of *dis*-continuity that we have today is the result of a historical anomaly, that is the period of the progressive welfarism of the post-war era. The echoes of the past that we hear, however, should not surprise us.

The nature of laws surrounding the question of poverty in society are not *only* particular to each historical circumstance throughout the history of capitalism – although they are partly that. Their *essential* logic stems from the nature of capitalism itself. We can therefore only understand poverty, and responses made to poverty, over the course of modern history by seeing it in terms of the essential form of exploitation which defines capitalism as well as the class structure and forms of class struggle associated with it.

In the history of capitalism poverty has been both a necessity and a problem to be solved. It has been a necessity for capitalists and their political functionaries in the sense of providing a constant reminder to productively employed workers of the consequences of losing their employment. It has been a problem to capitalism in the sense of the constant possibility it produces of riot and rebellion which has the potential to generalize throughout the whole of society. The tension between these two pressures has provided a focus for class struggle around the question of poverty. On the one hand, capitalists have in different epochs attempted to shape the nature and experience of poverty to suit their needs. On the other hand, it has been resistance by the poor themselves which has frustrated capitalists in this attempt and which has periodically forced them to retreat on the issue.

Our starting point must be the fact that the history of poverty *is* the history of capitalism. Of course there had been want and those who needed support from their communities before capitalism. Under Saxon law those who had no home of their own had to be taken in by those who had room. But when crops failed under feudalism the vulnerable simply starved, a fact to which the numerous famines of the Middle Ages, such as the one of 1315–17 in England, can testify. But poverty as a *mass* phenomenon and as a more or less constant and regularly appearing fact of life can be traced to the rise of capitalism.

Poverty and the Poor Laws in the late Middle Ages

What distinguished the social system of the late Middle Ages and the 'early modern era' was more than simply poverty; it was a very clear poverty-increasing tendency. It was not merely the numerical extent of poverty at that time, nor its near ubiquity, that lent it special importance, but its role in the formation of a new system: capitalism.

> The mediaeval perception of poverty had ... involved a particular kind of functionalism, and in the ideology of that time poverty had a specific role to play. Now, as the huge mass of beggars began to impinge on the collective consciousness, poverty came to be perceived as harmful to the public good. ... At the same time, however, the impoverishment of small producers had a new role to play, for it was a condition of the development of capitalism and an integral part of the first accumulation of capital. ... Thus poverty retained an important function in society, but the nature of this function had changed.
>
> (Geremek 1997: 102)

With the break up of the feudal estates in England during the fourteenth and fifteenth centuries, society began to change in a very fundamental way. As pasture and animal husbandry – particularly the grazing of sheep – replaced crops a major shift occurred towards less labour intensive methods of production. Peasants became increasingly transformed into waged land labourers. With the breakdown of the old feudal relationships of custom and obligation the phenomenon of mass rural unemployment in times of trade depression became more frequent. As money became increasingly important the 'cash-nexus' began to shape economic and social relationships. Consumables, chiefly food and clothing, became commodities for the first time. The age of pauperism had begun and with it came attempts by the state to control its impact on society and on economic relations.

The 'labour question' became an issue of state policy for the first time in the mid-fourteenth century. The impact of the first of the great plagues in 1349, which resulted in the massive depopulation of large parts of the country, greatly enhanced the bargaining position of the peasant. The labour shortage allowed the peasant, albeit unlawfully, to leave the manor to which he and his family had been bonded for as long as anyone could remember, confident in the knowledge that he could find work on a neighbouring estate. Wages rose sharply – increasing twofold, even threefold – over this period. The state was not slow to respond, however. In 1349 the ordinance decreed by the King's Council sought to legislate the wages which labourers could expect for certain types of work. In 1351 Parliament gave its support along with further elaboration of what this meant. The statute was nothing if not precise. It laid down the payment that could be asked for every type of work: hay could be mown for 5d an acre and a quarter of wheat could be threshed for 2½d. Every craft – carpentry, metalwork, stonemasonry, tailoring, etc. – was regulated in a similar manner.

> carters, ploughmen, leaders of the plough, shepherds, swineherds, domestic and all other servants shall receive the liveries and wages accustomed in the said twentieth year [of the reign of Edward III] and four years previously; so that in areas where wheat used to be given, they shall take 10d. for the bushel, or wheat at the will of the giver, unless it is ordained otherwise.
>
> (Dobson 1983: 64)

The Statute of Labourers cast a shadow over the lives of the peasantry and rural labourers for the next thirty years. It was returned to time and again by Parliament to be updated and refined. The giving of alms to vagabonds was outlawed. In 1360 a new statute was introduced which was designed to control the mobility of labour. Those who were found seeking work beyond the boundaries set for them were to have the letter 'F' for 'falsehood' branded on their foreheads. Further acts of Parliament sought to regulate the consumption of the poor – the Sumptuary laws of 1363 – which anticipated similar legislation under Edward IV and Henry VIII. The types of clothing and diet that could be enjoyed by the lower orders were set out in detail:

> Carters, ploughmen, drivers of the plough, oxherds, cowherds, shepherds, dairyworkers, and all other keepers of beasts, threshers of corn … shall not take or wear any manner of cloth but blanket and russet wool of 12d, and shall wear girdles of linen according to their estate, and come to eat and drink as in the manner that pertain to them and not excessively.
>
> (Jewell 1990: 67)

The clear message here is that the rising confidence of the feudal labourer had to be quelled. The Poor Laws of the fourteenth century represented a concerted attempt by the rulers of the day to reinstate the subdued condition of the peasantry which had prevailed before the plague of 1349. They were to become the site of a new form of class struggle as peasants pushed back against not only the exploitation of the manor but also the power of national state institutions. This gave rise to an increasingly generalized class consciousness as hatred of the penalties of the Statute of Labourers became focused on the richest in the land.

The social history of the fourteenth century is dominated by stories of vagrancy, truculent labour, strikes and combination between labourers on the manorial estates:

> The villeins appear to have shown such an ugly temper and such a determination to resist, that the bailiffs and master had to appeal to Parliament for force to support their rights. … 'Complaint has been made by the lords of the manors … that the villeins on their estates affirm them to be quite and utterly discharged of all manner of serfage … and will not suffer any distress or other justice to be made upon them; but do menace the ministers of their lords of life and member, and, which more is, gather themselves together in great routs and agree by such confederacy that everyone shall aid other to resist their lords with strong hand: and much other harm they do in sundry manner to the great damage of their said lords and evil example to others to begin such riots, so that, if due remedy be not the rather provided upon the same rebels, great mischief, which God prohibit, may thereof spring through the realm.'
>
> (Trevelyan 1972: 193–4)

'Great mischief' did indeed 'spring through the realm' only four years after these words were written with the outbreak of the Peasants' Revolt of 1381.

By the sixteenth century the process of disintegration of the feudal system was far more advanced. Wage labour was an increasingly dominant feature of the rural economy. The cloth industry in particular was the largest single employer after agriculture (Pound 1971: 7). The cycles of boom and slump and the consequent periods of unemployment associated with such industries produced a new pattern of periodic social unrest. During periods when unemployment struck, rioting, such as that at Lavenham and Sudbury in 1525, was usually not slow to follow. Land labourers who now fell on hard times could not rely on the protection of a manor. The enclosure of pasture for the ever expanding wool industry further reduced the amount of cultivated land available to the poor. A major contributory factor to the misery of the poor was the dissolution of the monasteries by Henry VIII. In 1536 the smaller abbeys and religious houses were dissolved and this was followed by the larger monasteries three years later. For centuries these had provided some shelter and sustenance for the destitute. With the removal of this support mass vagrancy assumed an altogether more dangerous form. Taxation records of the 1520s show that somewhere between one-third and a half of the population were very close to malnutrition (Beier 1983: 5). Along with vagrancy came begging, crime, social disorder and subversion. The preamble to the Public Relief Act 1531 complains that:

> in all places throughout this realm, vagabonds and beggars have of long time increased, and daily do increase in great and excessive numbers, by the occasion of idleness, mother and root of all vices bringing about continual thefts, murders and other heinous offences.
>
> (Nicholls 1898: I115)

Once again the response of the Tudor ruling class in the form of the acts of 1531 and 1536 reveal a great deal about the emergence of capitalism and the increasingly important role of 'free' waged labour. They also show a growing concern with the poor as a threat. The risings in Suffolk in 1525 had been provoked by taxes to fund the French wars and had involved large numbers of the destitute cloth workers. They were followed two years later by serious disturbances in Norwich and Great Yarmouth. Of particular concern were the mariners and militiamen recently returned from the continent. These men were trained in arms and their entry into the ranks of the poor posed a genuine threat to the authorities. It was men like these who would much later, in 1589, occupy the City of London for several days. The period was also marked by political instability. This was especially apparent during the years of the minority of Edward VI. The presence of a boy king on the throne led to political opportunism and factionalism and the poor were easy recruits for rebel armies got up by rebel leaders. It was this fear of subversion that informed much of thinking behind the Poor Laws of the time. In the words of a Yorkshire Justice of the Peace:

> To stay the spreading of false and seditious rumours and the sending of messages from the late rebels to trouble the quiet of the realm, order is to be given in market towns and other places that all suspected passengers, vagabonds, beggars and rogues be punished with the severity and celerity, according to the late statute.
>
> (Pound 1971: 46)

The Poor Law Acts of the early sixteenth century stand out for three reasons. We can see the first acknowledgement of a role for the state in the care of the infirm. Local officials were obliged for the first time to provide support for the elderly and 'impotent'. There was also an obligation on the state to provide work for the able-bodied poor and for provision to be made for destitute children. The use of the term 'care' should be taken advisedly. The conditions provided for the infirm, when they were provided at all, were grim. And the situation for children taken into homes was little better than slavery. These pieces of legislation are also remarkable for the severity of the punishments given for infringements by those deemed fit to work. These were years in which local Justices of the Peace were given even greater powers of punishment for vagrancy and begging. Those who were caught offending could be tied to carts and dragged through the town, whipped until they were bloody, have the 'gristle' part of their ears cut off, be branded on their face or breast and, for the most unreformable, be hanged.

Finally, we should note the much more pronounced distinction which was made between the 'deserving' and the 'undeserving' poor. This distinction became essential as the state, concerned at the destabilizing effect of large-scale pauperism, saw the necessity of providing some measure of support for the very poorest. At the same time, however, there was a concern that poverty should not be seen as an 'option' by the working poor. Apart from the ferocious humiliation inflicted on those who begged without license, there were specifically proscribed occupations by which the non-working poor might make ends meet, such as fortune-telling, palmistry and other 'crafty science'.

In 1563 further legislation cast the terms of poor relief very clearly in the form of a labour policy. The Statute of Artificers and Compulsory Assessment of that year set the minimum duration of employment with a master at one year. Householders were authorized to take in the unemployed as 'apprentices' for up to seven years. Justices of the Peace could order anybody, even already employed labourers, to work in the fields at harvest time. Wage levels were set as were hours of work and even meal times. Further restrictions were imposed on the ability of labourers to travel to look for work. In previous epochs, despite the oppressions of feudalism, it was possible for a peasant to enjoy at least a modicum of independence by virtue of the fact that he might work his own land. But, as Marx states,

> What the capitalist system demanded was the reverse of this: a degraded and almost servile condition of the mass of the people, their transformation into mercenaries, and the transformation of their means of labour into capital.
>
> (Marx 1988 [1867]: 880–1)

There was a point to this deliberate and organized humiliation of the poor. The economic basis of society was changing. Capitalist relations of production were not simply emerging side by side with feudalism as an alternative to be switched to at a time of political crisis. Rather, the new commercialism was permeating all aspects of life and was affecting all economic and productive activity in the rural areas as well as in the towns. It had been necessary to detach the labourer from the land in a specific sense – no labourer was to feel an affinity with a *particular* piece of land. Similarly, no specific relationship of duties and obligations should exist between a labourer and any particular landowner. The figure of the 'free' worker was emerging on to the historical landscape.

For the capitalist this provided a flexibility which allowed the shedding of labour during the winter or in times of trade depression. But it also opened up options to the labourer when times were good. Travelling from town to town for work could be a more attractive option than being tied down to one employer. Casual work and begging provided a marginal livelihood but none the less one that meant an escape from the petty discipline of the master's overseer. It was options like these, from the capitalists' point of view, that had to be closed down as while they existed it was all the more difficult to force labourers to accept low wages and poor working conditions. Employers could no longer appeal to workers on the basis of loyalty or custom, and, in principle, any worker could work for any employer. The discipline the labourer had now to be forced to accept could no longer draw on historical family ties. The relationship between the two sides had become an immediate one and was dominated by money. The point of the Poor Laws of the sixteenth century was to strengthen the coercive reality which was concealed behind the facade of the 'freedom' of the relationship between labourer and employer. The century that was to follow, however, was a century of revolution and the question of poverty was now cast in an altogether different light.

The turn of the century saw the introduction of more Poor Laws. The legislation of 1598 and its elaboration in 1601 was notable for its emphasis on family responsibility. Parents were responsible not only for their children but also for grandparents who couldn't look after themselves. Children whose families could not support them were to be taken as apprentices until the age of 24, in the case of males, and until the age of 21, in the case of females. The family was also responsible for any of its members who were incapacitated due to injury or a medical condition, such as blindness. The dissolving of the manorial communities of the medieval world had swept away the reciprocal relationship between landowner and labourer which the infirm had traditionally been able to fall back on. The emphasis on the role of the family as the primary social unit of care, thus freeing the state of the burden of supporting the needy, dates from this period and became a definitive feature of the social response to poverty under capitalism which survives to this present day. The Poor Law Acts of the seventeenth century also saw the strengthening of the powers of local Justices of the Peace who had the special responsibility of administrating and implementing these laws. We see this strengthening of the local state in conjunction with almost every new piece of legislation concerning the poor from this point onwards.

The new attitude to the poor was now finding a much more developed and ideological expression in the thinking of people who were to have a great influence on some of the chief protagonists of the English Civil War. Christopher Hill (1994), in his book *Puritanism and Revolution*, pays particular attention to William Perkins, and his discussion is useful to us here. Perkins articulated what Hill calls a 'transvaluation' which occurred from the late medieval period to his own time on the question of the poor. The surplus of the lord of the manor was not invested in the way that the profit of the capitalists was to be. Rather, the lord and his family would either consume the surplus or use it in various ways to secure the allegiance and fealty of society around them. This often took the form of patronage and charity in times of want. The status of the lord and the esteem in which he was held was determined, in part, by the support he gave to the needy. Charity was a virtue. For the capitalist, as we have seen, the notion of unconditional support for the poor was considered wrong, and was viewed as undermining the social discipline required by the new system. Charity was a vice.

> Indiscriminate alms-giving by the rich man in his castle had yielded place to a careful search for the industrious or impotent poor conducted by bourgeois churchwardens. Conspicuous waste has ceased to be a social obligation and is regarded as an anti-social vice. The sordid sin of avarice has been transmuted into the religious and patriotic duty of thrift. Whereas in 1500 the businessman 'had practised extortion and been told that it was wrong; for it was contrary to the law of God' he was now 'told that it was right; for it was in accordance with the law of nature'.
>
> (Hill 1994: 198)

The ideology developed by the puritans on the question of poverty was only one half of the picture, however. The other was the response of the poor themselves. This was to become a crucial factor in the course of the Civil War. There was hostility to the new teaching of people such as Perkins from the outset. As the century wore on, this hostility took a more active form. As Hill explains, there were 'Levellers' in Northamptonshire in 1607 and 'Diggers' in Warwickshire. Serious revolts by the poor occurred in the south-west of England in 1628–31, and there were widespread movements against enclosure in 1640–3 – the early years of the revolution. Thus by the time of the Civil War there was a 'steady undercurrent of fear of the "many-headed monster" ' of class struggle (Hill, C. 1993: 21). Large-scale riots and disturbances were occurring against the background of a depression in the trades, especially in the cloth industry. The social character of these movements was that 'weavers and artisans seem to have predominated ... with a sprinkling of husbandmen and yeomen' (Manning 1996: 49).

The contradiction of the position of the puritans now became clear. On the one hand their ideology dictated a harsh attitude towards the poor. As a contemporary observer put it, 'The only riches of a commonwealth is by employing the poor and making such industrious as are not' (quoted in Slack 1988: 30). On the other hand, they were making a revolution in which the poor were playing a decisive role. Indeed, the poor gave to the revolution its radical democratic content. The parliamentarians needed the support of the poor to carry their revolution through to a successful outcome, and one consequence of this was that they discovered a new-found generosity. Pamphlets appeared urging anti-poverty measures that were friendly towards the poor. In addition, in 1647, the London Corporation of the Poor, a body concerned with the welfare of the poorest in society, was founded. Hill argues that the poor were better off in the 1650s than in any other previous decade (Hill, C. 1993: 131). With the end of the Civil War, however, and the defeat of the radicals, the puritan ideology and the new capitalist attitude towards the poor once again became dominant.

After the Civil War the main concern of subsequent Poor Law legislation was the restriction of the mobility of the poor. The new puritan ideology of work for the poor and thrift for the rich could not be imposed effectively if labourers could up and leave as the mood took them. The 'freedom' of the wage labourer had to be gutted of any real content beyond its merely ideological form. One contemporary observer commented ironically:

> In a free nation where slaves are not allowed of, the surest wealth consists in a multitude of laborious poor. ... To make the society happy and people easy under the meanest circumstances, it is necessary that great numbers of them should be ignorant as well as poor. ... We have hardly poor enough to do what is necessary to make us subsist. ... Men who are to remain and end their days in laborious, tiresome and painful station of life, the sooner they are put upon it, the more patiently they'll submit to it for ever after.
>
> (quoted in Hill, C. 1993: 229)

The Poor Relief Act 1662 became known as the Settlement Act. It allowed local Justices of the Peace to remove any labourer who had arrived in their area within the previous forty days to the place from whence they had come. There was a particular concern to keep the poor away from the cities. The provisions of the 1662 Act were intensified towards the end of the century with the introduction of the Act for Supplying Some Defects in the Law for the Relief of the Poor of this Kingdom. Under this Act of 1697 magistrates were given greater powers of removal. It also added the element of conspicuous humiliation of the poor. All those who received poor relief, including children, had to wear a letter 'P' in blue sewn into their clothing as a public mark of their condition. Those who 'chose' poverty were to be reduced to a miserable station in life. It was only with the whiff of revolution once again that the establishment of the late eighteenth century were to modify their approach towards the poor.

The later decades of the 1700s are marked by episodes of political crisis for the establishment in Britain. Widespread radical agitation in England occurred at the time of the American War of Independence and tension was high within ruling circles. Pamphlets such as the one written by John Cartwright, entitled *Take Your Choice*, urged universal suffrage and the extension of political rights in a manner which anticipated the Chartist movement of the nineteenth century. Other agitations such as the 'Wilkes and Liberty' campaign around the MP John Wilkes aimed towards similar goals. Throughout the 1780s food rioting was recurrent. Even the Gordon Riots of 1780, which had begun as reactionary anti-Catholic riots, became an opportunity for a more widespread disaffection to explode throughout London. The riots ended with the burning down of the Newgate prison at St Paul's.

It was the impact of the French Revolution of 1789, however, and the spread of English Jacobinism, that forced the ruling class to rethink their attitude towards the poor. The prospect of a major revolt from below was to produce a mellowing of the more punitive aspects of the English Poor Laws as well as a restructuring of poor relief on a fundamental level. By the 1790s the radical agitations which had begun in the 1770s had assumed a much more working-class, artisan character. Disturbances had become much more serious, as had establishment fears of a revolution. In 1795 catastrophic harvests led to food scarcity and widespread rioting. In October of that year, 200,000 people turned out on the occasion of the King's opening of Parliament. As the King's procession went by his coach was attacked. The crowd booed and hissed and cries of 'Bread! Peace! Peace!' went up. The state attempted to clamp down on the subversion. The London Corresponding Society, the earliest of the working-class political reform societies, was repressed; the Treasonable Practices Act and the Seditious Meetings Act were both passed. The fear of the poor, however, continued.

In 1795 a group of Justices of the Peace met at Speenhamland, Berkshire. They decided to ameliorate the condition of the labourers with a system of wage supplementation. The system was made law in the Poor Relief Act of the same year. This Act in effect represented a return to a form of outdoor relief – the provision of relief to the labourer in his home – which had been abandoned by the Act of 1722. The Speenhamland system was to become a hated form of poor relief because of the effect it was to have in depressing wages. Farmers presumed that they could lower wages and that their labourers would have their incomes supplemented by the parish. None the less, against the background of revolution on the continent and the spirit of hunger and revolt in England, Speenhamland did represent a retreat by the establishment in the face of an increasingly restive working popula-tion. The following puts it well:

> There was a special reason why the classes that had suddenly become very much richer should dread too searching a discontent at this moment. They had seen titles and all seigniorial dues abol-ished almost at a single stroke across the Channel, and they were at this time associating constantly with the emigrant nobility of France. ... The richer classes ... were naturally anxious to soothe and pacify the poor before discontent spread any further.
> (Hammond and Hammond 1995: 168–9)

The Speenhamland system was to last forty years before being replaced by legislation that directly reflected the interests of an ascendant and world conquering English capitalist class. But it was also this legislation that would provoke the most serious working-class reaction seen up until that point in English social history, in the form of a powerful and sustained anti-Poor Law movement. It was to be a movement which also contributed to a rising and developing independent working-class consciousness.

The 'new' Poor Law

The coming to power of the Whigs in 1830 was seen as heralding a new age and a new consensus within British politics. Workers generally saw in the Whigs the possibility of progress, particularly with regard to the question of the vote. The Whigs themselves had campaigned on the basis of suffrage reform and on their election to government they set about honouring this promise. In 1831 the Reform Bill which sought to extend the vote to the middle classes caused enormous excitement throughout the country. This excitement built into a frenzy as workers began to feel that they also might soon benefit from this new beginning. Some measure of how high feelings were running is given in the fact that severe rioting broke out in Bristol when an anti-reform figure tried to enter the town. On that occasion peace was restored only after four days of fighting with troops. These high hopes, however, despite the passing of the 1832 Reform Act, were soon to be smashed.

The Whigs did indeed represent a new consensus within British society. But it was not one in which workers were to share. The new consensus among the capitalist class and their newly won allies in the middle and petty commercial classes was aimed *against* the working class of the 1830s. The 1830s saw the zenith of the Industrial Revolution. These were the years which witnessed the building of the canals and railways, the breathless expansion of the textile mills and an increasingly industrial horizon. The question of the response of the working poor to these events as well as the question of labour discipline had taken on a new and unprecedented urgency. The ferocity of the Whigs' attitudes and policies towards the poor directly reflected the new situation.

There are two fronts on which the Whigs moved which are relevant to our theme. First, they attacked the general union movement which had swept through the industrial regions. Robert Owen's Grand National Consolidated Trade Union had mushroomed from a few thousand members at the beginning of 1834 to over 700,000 by the summer. The Whigs reacted with imprisonment and deportations, for example the Dorchester labourers of Tolpuddle fame and the leaders of the Glasgow cotton spinners, who were later to play an important role in the working-class movement when they returned from exile. These were measures to which the working-class movement at that point had no response. The general union movement collapsed after a few glorious months which had proved the ability of the workers to organize along lines of class rather than craft.

The second line of attack from the Whigs against the working class was on the front of Poor Law reform. For the government the *cost* of poor relief was certainly an issue. The industrial system which they celebrated, and which had brought the new industrialists their fortunes, was fast creating a pauperized working class. Each month thousands of destitute folk were streaming into the cities from the rural areas. The rapid cycles of the new system produced violent downturns of production and thousands of workers were thrown out of their employment in the mills, factories and mines. Poor relief throughout the 1830s hovered between £6–7 million (Marshall 1968: 26–7), an amount the Whigs were determined to reduce.

However, there was another much more fundamental theme underlying the thinking of the Whigs and the capitalists from where they drew most of their support. The problem with Speenhamland for the

Whigs was not just that it had represented a retreat at a time of revolutionary crisis, but that it was too extensive and, in their view, too generous. In allowing the unemployed worker the dignity of his or her independence, allowing poor relief to be paid at the home, they saw no deterrence from idleness. For the new industrial system to work, for workers to accept the barrack-like regimes of the mills and the payment of starvation wages, they had to be made totally dependent on the capitalist for work. Once again unemployment could not be seen as an 'option'. Poverty had to be experienced and seen as an utterly degraded condition. In the words of Lord Althorpe, speaking for the bill, poverty had to be experienced as a 'misfortune' and anything which detracted from this had to be eliminated (Nicholls 1898: ii267). Sir George Nicholls, himself one of the commissioners, put it more bluntly:

> I wish to see the Poor House looked to with dread by the labour-
> ing classes, and the reproach for being an inmate of it extend
> down from father to son. ... For without this, where is the stimu-
> lus to industry?
>
> (Quoted in Novak 1988: 47)

The possibility of losing one's job had to be seen to be a terrifying thing if the wheels of the new industrial machines were to keep turning out the handsome profits of capitalist exploitation. The 'problem', complained the commissioners' report, was that the old Poor Law was not ruthless enough:

> The labourer feels that the existing system, though it gives him low
> wages, always gives him easy work. It gives him also, strange as it
> may appear, what he values more, a sort of independence. He
> need not bestir himself to please his master; he need not put any
> restraint on his temper; he need not ask for relief as a favour. He
> has all the slave's security for subsistence without his liability to
> punishment.
>
> (Quoted in Novak 1988: 44)

This, then, was the background to the Poor Law Amendment Act of 1834.

The chief ideological support for the new Poor Law came from Malthus and Bentham. Whilst Malthus had warned against support for the poor on the basis of catastrophic predictions about the dangers of overpopulation, Bentham preached the virtues of a centralized rational administration and the throwing out of the social relics of feudalism. Speenhamland, then, with its support for the unemployed worker and his family and its quaint variations from parish to parish, was to be swept aside to make way for the austere regime of the workhouse. Bentham also had a more direct influence through one of his disciples, Edwin Chadwick, one of the authors of the new Poor Law. Bentham had put forward the principle of 'less eligibility', according to which poor relief should be set at below the level of income of the worst paid. This also applied to general conditions and diet:

> Only the cheapest fare should be served in the house; an ample fare might be served only if it did not 'render the condition of the burdensome poor more desirable than that of the self-maintaining poor'.
>
> (Quoted in Cowherd 1977: 93)

This principle found its way into the bill. Once again, unemployment could not be allowed to become an 'option' for the poor. Equally, the rural poor had to be forced into the cities. Even after being driven off the land by enclosure or, as is more likely by this period, thrown out of work by a depression in agriculture, rural labourers generally preferred to survive as best they could outside of the towns on parish relief rather than enter the textile mills in the industrial north. The abolition of out-relief cut away this support. The introduction of a workhouse in a rural area was often swiftly followed by carts which came to transport the destitute of the farming areas into the hands of the factory overseer. The poor had to work at whatever rates of pay the employers chose and poor relief was to work on the terms set by the new industrial system.

At the same time, activities which softened the sting of poverty were being steadily eroded. Working-class customs and leisure pursuits that harked back to earlier times were suppressed by Acts of Parliament. As land became enclosed, hunting for game for the table became *poaching*. Locations for outdoor entertainments were restricted as more and more land was designated private. This led to struggles for access to common land, such as the successful fight over the right of access to Epping Forest. In 1820 a concerted campaign took place against the working-class fair (Cunningham 1980: 25). The message was that poverty was to be *suffered*, not enjoyed. The introduction of the workhouses was a central part of this new social discipline.

From their inception the workhouses were feared and hated by the working class. The new 'Bastilles', as they were called, came to represent the profoundly anti-working-class stance of the Whig government. The new Poor Laws had done away with out-relief. Now the unemployed worker would have to sacrifice his or her freedom if they wished to seek support from the state and enter the workhouse. The regimes inside the workhouses were dreadful. Husbands and wives were separated, children were taken from their mothers, the healthy were put together with the diseased. The main element of psychological deterrence in the union workhouse was its system of classifying inmates. Labourers in Cambridgeshire stated in a petition to Parliament in 1836 that they were

> dismayed and disgusted beyond anything they can describe, with the idea of being shut up in one part of a prison and their wives and children in other separate parts because they are poor through no fault of their own.

> (Digby 1982: 17)

Inmates were immediately set to work performing arduous and degrading tasks: mending sacks and picking oakum – pulling the threads of old rope – were common workhouse tasks. Once somebody had become an inmate of the workhouse they were very unlikely ever to leave. The destitute went to the workhouse to die. It is no wonder that workers refused to take the workhouse test. A person had to be beyond hope to finally give themselves up to the workhouse system.

In the 1840s a series of scandals brought to the attention of the wider public the true picture of what was going on inside the workhouses. The most famous of these was at the Andover workhouse in 1846. Inmates had been given bones to grind and vicious fighting broke out over the putrid scraps of meat that were stuck to the bones. Similar scandals occurred at Eversholt, Bridgewater, Sevenoaks and Keithly.

The anti-Poor Law movement

A movement against the workhouse began just over a year after the bill was passed, with hundreds of petitions being collected from all over the country. In May 1837 a mass rally against the Poor Laws was held at Hartshead moor near Leeds. At least 100,000 (the figure is probably nearer 200,000) turned out to hear speakers condemn the Act. The demonstration formed as local processions flowed into a greater and greater assemblage. Each of the different processions carried their own colours and banners. Bands were interspersed throughout the demonstration and something of a carnival atmosphere prevailed at the moor, with refreshments being served. But it was not merely the impressive display of organization and discipline which unnerved the authorities. It was also the detectable undertone of violent and uncompromising opposition to everything that the new Poor Law represented. The colours that were carried give some indication of the underlying mood. One flag showed three hanging figures, and the inscription below read: 'The three Poor Law Commissioners drawing their wages'. The Huddersfield section proudly led the demonstration with their banner which declared: 'The Huddersfield division swears destruction to all Malthusian bastilles' (Knott 1986: 114–16). If the point needed driving home, then it was when the editor of the pro-new Poor Law newspaper, the *Leeds Mercury*, expressed his contempt for the demonstration. His effigy was burned all over the West Ridings, and at York it was carried around on a donkey for public ridicule before being shot (ibid.: 123).

The movement was strongest in the northern regions – Leeds, Bradford and Huddersfield – but it was occurring in many other counties as well, such as Kent, Cheshire, Carlisle and Norfolk. New workhouses in the process of being built were torn down brick by brick or were torched. Guardians of the Poor Law were physically attacked. The movement was beginning to assume an insurrectionary air. Major bloody confrontations took place between workers and troops attempting to defend workhouses. In Kent things took a peculiar turn when a man declaring himself to be the Messiah led a semi-religious movement against the new Poor Law. The Kent movement was finally put down when its leader was killed by troops, and several members of the crowd were felled by gunfire. Large riots took place in Bradford, Huddersfield, Dewsbury and Todmorden. In the West Ridings, Poor Law guardians, and one in particular, Assistant Commissioner Alfred Power, came to fear for their lives as their every public appearance became an occasion for disturbance and riot. By the summer of 1837 'The crowd had done its work and needed to do no more; the mere threat of violence was enough to keep the pro-Poor Law Guardians away or inactive' (Edsall 1971: 98). The effect of the movement was to slow down the implementation of the new Poor Law. There were many areas in which the new regime could not be implemented, and by 1836 it was only operating in sixty-four localities (Rothstein 1929: 32).

The movement's potential for violence posed a serious threat to the authorities. As Cobbett predicted in his *Political Register* in 1834: 'If this bill be attempted to be put into execution, there will be a revolution in England.' A year later he described the atmosphere in the northern regions:

> Half a dozen counties are in a state of partial commotion; the jails are opening the doors to receive those who are called the rebels against the Poor-Law bill. No matter as to any other thing relative to this measure; here is the country; disturbed; here are the jails filling; here are the housewives and children screaming after their fathers; here are the undeniable facts.
>
> (Quoted in Brown and Daniels 1984: 24)

Feargus O'Connor, who was to become the most nationally important figure to lead the Chartist movement, toured the northern industrial districts. Everywhere he went he established Radical Associations which advocated the repeal of the new Poor Law. In many cases the anti-Poor Law committees, which were springing up all over the West Ridings and beyond, evolved directly from the 'short-time' committees which had campaigned for the shortening of the working day. This process of the coalescence of movements was an important development: the consciousness of workers was shifting towards a much more generalized opposition to the social structure itself.

Several important spokesmen began to emerge who articulated the revulsion felt by workers at the new system. In Parliament Fielden made powerful speeches against the workhouse and called for factory reform and the reduction of the working day. By far the most influential figure, however, and the person who really captured the feelings of the working class, was the Methodist minister, the Reverend Raynor Stephens. Stephens' rhetoric caught the general discontent of the working class and infused it with an Old Testament fury:

> And if this damnable law, which violated all the laws of God, was continued, and all means of peaceably putting an end to it had been made in vain, then, in the words of their banner, 'For children and wife we'll war to the knife'. If the people who produce all wealth could not be allowed, according to God's word, to have the kindly fruits of the earth which they had, in obedience to God's Word, raised by the sweat of their brow, then war to the knife

with their enemies, who were the enemies of God. If the musket and the pistol, the sword and the pike were to no avail, let the woman take the scissors, the child the pin and needle. If all failed, then the firebrand – aye, the firebrand, I repeat. The palace shall be in flames.

(Quoted in Brown and Daniels 1984: 24)

And in a speech at Newcastle he proclaimed:

Newcastle ought to be and should be one blaze of fire, with only one way to put it out, and that with the blood of all who supported this abominable measure ... and let every man with a torch in one hand and a dagger in the other, put to death any and all who attempted to sever man and wife.

(Quoted in Hopkins 1979: 93)

Richard Oastler and other figures spoke in a similar vein:

CHRISTIAN READER
Be not alarmed at the sound of the Title. I cannot bless that which GOD and NATURE CURSE. The Bible being true, the Poor Law Amendment Act is false! The Bible contains the will of God – this accursed Act of Parliament embodies the will of Lucifer. It is the Sceptre of Belial, establishing its sway in the land of Bibles!! DAMNATION; ETERNAL DAMNATION TO THE ACCURSED FIEND!

(Quoted in Hopkins 1979: 93)

Some of the key names of the period addressed this new movement of the working class: Feargus O'Connor, Robert Owen, Henry Hetherington, James Bronterre O'Brien, Reverend Stephens, Richard Oastler. It is no surprise that several of these people later went on to play important, and mostly heroic, roles in the Chartist movement. For what was happening was more than merely a single campaign against one Act of Parliament. Several campaigns of the working class – the anti-Poor Law campaign, the struggle for a free press, the short-time campaign to reduce the length of the working day, the struggle for free trade unions – were coalescing into a generalized consciousness of the working class. For the first time, the industrial working class was raising itself in its own eyes into a position to stand full square against an establishment which had previously put it down. The anti-Poor Law movement soon went into decline, but this happened only when its energies became channelled into a movement which took the working class to a new level of social and political struggle.

Conclusion

By 1838 it was clear to many thousands of workers that to campaign against the new Poor Law in isolation from the other issues that the Whigs were throwing at the working class was to fight at a disadvantage. A general consensus emerged that the problem was not simply factory conditions, or the workhouse system, or even the Whigs themselves. Rather, it was the very nature of a political system which excluded the working class from any effective power or influence. All of the various campaigns and battles fought by workers over the previous half decade now flowed into the Chartist movement for political emancipation. For some moderates within the movement, such as Place and Lovett, the launch of the Charter represented an attempt to curb the violence of the anti-Poor Law movement. But if the intellectual leadership of Chartism, as well as the nuclei of local organization, had come from such campaigns as those conducted against the newspaper tax and for the ten-hour working day, the popular energy and revolutionary fervour of the early Chartist movement undoubtedly came from the struggle against the workhouse. At high points of Chartist agitation the issue of the new Poor Law often found expression in the rhetoric of leaders and in the actions of workers themselves. A symbolic moment of the 1842 general strike was the attacking of the Stockport workhouse and the liberation of its inmates.

The Poor Law Amendment Act of 1834 was in effect an attempt to impose a once and for all settlement of the question of the poor on the capitalists' terms. Poverty was a *necessity* for the new system. It existed as a threat to the working class. If workers were to be made to accept the horrors of the factory system then unemployment and the poverty consequent upon it had to be, and had to be *seen* to be, a terrible thing, something that nobody but the most desperate and defeated could contemplate. The highly visible workhouse buildings, along with their cousins the debtors' prisons, were to act as constant reminders of this fact. In all of this the Poor Law guardians of the 1830s were carrying on and taking to a new height a theme which had characterized capitalism from its earliest beginnings in the break up of the medieval system. The labour statutes of the fourteenth century, the Poor Laws of the Tudor period and the punishment of poverty under the puritan legislation of the decades following the Civil War all prefigured the logic of the 1834 Act.

However, if capitalism needed poverty to impose its economic and social discipline, it also had to contend with the response of the poor themselves. Over various periods of time – in 1381 with the Peasants' Revolt, during the English Civil War, in the period of the radical and working-class agitation of the 1790s and with the anti-Poor Law movement of the 1830s and the rise of the first political working-class movement, Chartism, – the poor threatened their rulers with revolution and forced them to retreat. In each phase of this historical theme the details of the story have varied according to the particular historical context and to the level of capitalist development. The underlying logic, however, has represented a historical continuity and does so still today.

Today we see a new chapter of this story unfolding in Britain with the welfare reform policies of the New Labour government. The arguments which the government uses to justify its 'reforms' and its ideology with respect to the poor draw on some long-standing and even ancient prejudices. The 'modern' it seems is not so modern after all. The ongoing schizophrenia and oscillation between using poverty as a stick to hold over the working class on the one hand, and the constant danger for the ruling class of revolts by the poor acting as a detonator for a wider class confrontation on the other, will remain. It is only the outcome we cannot predict.

3 Class struggle, self-help and popular welfare

Chris Jones and Tony Novak

Introduction

Welfare has always been at the heart of class struggle, or at least at the heart of the popular struggle from below. In the final analysis it is a concern for human welfare, rather than abstract notions of political or economic analysis, that has fuelled the struggle for social transformation. The vision of a better society based on social justice, that treats people equally, with tolerance and respect, has for centuries motivated millions in the fight for economic, social and political change. It is equally against the insecurities and inequalities of capitalism, its denial of welfare and its degradation of human spirit and well-being, that millions have struggled and will continue to do so.

This is not to say that the struggle has been directed towards, or satisfied with, the provision of those formal institutions of 'welfare' that are commonly associated with the welfare state. On the contrary, as Henry Pelling has argued,

> the extension of the power of the state at the beginning of this century which is generally regarded as having laid the basis of the welfare state was by no means welcomed by members of the working class, was indeed undertaken over the critical hostility of many of them, perhaps of most of them.
>
> (Pelling 1968: 2; see also Thane 1984)

Even at the height of its relatively short-lived history during the two or three decades that followed the Second World War, this so-called welfare state fell far short of meeting the needs and requirements of ordinary people. In its dealings with the poor, with women, black people and others it frequently gave with one hand what it took away with the other, reinforcing patterns of oppression as much as relieving them. Still less did it succeed in fundamentally challenging the principles and priorities of capitalist society, to create a society based on principles of human welfare rather than private profit. Caught between the contradictory demands of human welfare on the one hand, and a private enterprise economy on the other, at its best the welfare state offered a compromise, although one that was not to last. It mitigated, but never removed, the economic insecurities on which capitalism depends, providing some insurance against risks rather than removing the risk. As a large, critical social policy literature illustrates, the welfare state in Britain, as elsewhere, brought about a limited redistribution of resources – more in a horizontal than a vertical direction – that would leave the fundamental contours of wealth and poverty intact. What is more, while the state has responded to the growing demand for welfare, it has done so in a way that has all too often fragmented, divided and disarmed those who have demanded it.

Even in its limited and contradictory form, however, the welfare state proved, from the point of view of capital, too much of a compromise. Since then, the restructuring of welfare and the state that has taken place under both Conservative and New Labour governments since the late 1970s has seen state social policy retreat even further from a commitment to welfare. In its place have been re-established principles and practices of discipline and regulation of the poor that have historically been more familiar patterns of working-class experience of the state (Jones and Novak 1999).

The growth of state welfare in Britain at the beginning of the twentieth century to which Pelling refers in the above quotation was not of course an intervention into a vacuum. State intervention is always in a particular political context. In this case it was into a society where, by necessity, working people had already done what they could to protect themselves from the insecurities and poverty of capitalism, and to provide for themselves those things that the market could not or would not provide. During the course of the nineteenth century working people had established widespread formal and informal processes and institutions of welfare of their own to meet their needs. These included a vast network of friendly societies and savings clubs, working-class schools, food and other co-operatives and health societies, some highly organized and built into the structures of the trades union and labour movement, others much more local, informal and irregular.

State welfare in its expansion from the beginning of the twentieth century onwards was in many important respects to conflict with these alternative forms of popular welfare. It was not only that state welfare was to rival but also, as we shall see, that it was to seek to undermine, incorporate, or supplant its popular alternatives. During the course of the twentieth century, as state welfare expanded on an unprecedented scale, popular struggles over welfare were to be drawn increasingly into debate and involvement with the forms of welfare that the state provided. But while popular forms and models of welfare diminished from the height and scale which they had achieved in the nineteenth century, they nevertheless have continued to surface and thrive, offering a radical alternative to what the state has to offer.

These two, often conflicting, patterns of welfare provision – state welfare and popular welfare – form the focus of this chapter. We seek to rescue from historical and contemporary neglect the significance of popular self-help and welfare both as a political movement and as an example of welfare provision. In this sense, we argue for the importance of self-help as a prefigurative form of activity. Popular welfare offers a vision of how the world might be different, of how welfare might be organized and what it could mean. But it is also prefigurative in terms of creating the political practice that might contribute to the political movement necessary to enable that change to be brought about. At the same time, we argue that state welfare, in its encounters with its popular alternative, has continued not only to fall short of the socialist vision, but also has been directed in part to thwart its realization.

Self-help

We need first, however, to say something about the concepts which we use in this chapter. 'Self-help' is a politically ambiguous term. It has, especially in recent years, although not for the first time, been hijacked by the political right who have appropriated it to their own vision of individual selfishness and the absence of social institutions and mechanisms of support. Self-help has for a very long time been used by the establishment to argue that people should stand on their own feet, and not look to others for support. More recently it has been used to justify the dismantling even of that limited state welfare provision which is itself now seen as undermining individual effort and creating a dependency culture.

This association of self-help with the individualistic politics of the right perhaps explains why many on the left neglect its history and contemporary significance, or dismiss it, as Tom Nairn once did, as 'a caricature of bourgeois ultra-respectability' (Nairn 1972: 188). This depiction of working-class self-help, usually ascribed to the nineteenth-century labour aristocracy among whom it was most developed, as a process 'whereby bourgeois ideas and customs were refracted down into the working class' (ibid.) simply will not do. Working-class self-help is far too complex to be written off simply as a reflection of bourgeois ideas and values. Of course, there have been those within the working class who have lauded self-help in these terms, but there have equally been those who have seen it as essential to a successful workers' movement. Working-class self-help has never been a single activity or process but has always run along a continuum from an acceptance of the status quo and an attempt to secure a niche within it to a determined independence of working-class activity as a means to overcome it. While self-help did have its bourgeois counterparts, its roots within working-class culture and struggle signalled working-class self-help as a very different form of activity and political conscious-ness. It was rather, in the words of a leading pioneer of the co-operative movement, George Holyoake, one in which workers 'took their affairs into their own hands, and what is more to the point ... kept them in their own hands' (quoted in Bonner 1961: 41).

Whatever its bourgeois caricature might suggest, self-help was and remains an essential part of popular struggle, and has been fundamen-tal to the formation and development of the working-class movement. It was through working-class self-help during the course of the nineteenth century that the mass of people sought to protect them-selves against the threats of unemployment, sickness and old age, as well as a host of other problems which industrial capitalism brought in its wake. At their height the formal organizations of the Friendly Society Movement were alone to have over five million members – three times the membership of trades unions – to say nothing of the countless local and informal savings clubs, sickness and burial societies and other organizations through which people came together for their own mutual benefit. The co-operative movement was equally significant as a major source of working-class radicalism, and a symbol of the benefits of mutual aid over competitive individualism. To neglect this history of self-help, as well as its contemporary manifesta-tions, or to dismiss it on the basis of a specious claim of the right to have a monopoly on its definition, is thus to surrender what was once a central principle of working-class organization and struggle, and which continues to characterize struggles of the oppressed.

This notion of collective, independent and autonomous activity – the notion of self-help that we would employ – is not of course confined to 'working-class struggle' in the conventional sense. It is also evident in the struggles of the poor, of women, of black people, of disabled people and others. That many of these struggles revolve around welfare, around attempts to construct alternative models and practices in the face of a state system felt to be at best irrelevant and at worst opposed to what people want and need, should force us to sit up and take notice of what is going on.

To take but one example, one of the most significant of recent popular welfare initiatives has been the array of activities developed by gay men and lesbians in the face of the HIV/Aids pandemic. In both Britain and the USA, especially during the 1980s, the explicit homophobia of much of the establishment and state welfare agencies meant that those suffering from HIV/Aids were faced with victim-blaming, demonizing and inadequate services. In a classic reformulation of popular welfare, activists both denounced the inhumanity of official welfare and set about constructing their own alternative services. In such cities as London, Manchester, New York and San Francisco networks of advice, education and support were established by and within gay communities themselves. What characterized these initiatives was a fundamental respect for those who were suffering, and the attempt to create services based on what they themselves knew that they needed, rather than what the professionals said that they needed. In this example, the 'buddy' system of support for those with terminal illness marked a significant landmark in welfare provision, and constitutes the sort of prefigurative initiative that could inform the construction of alternative welfare provision.

Self-help and popular culture

For the most part people's welfare is not looked after or provided for in state institutions or via state welfare professionals and agencies, but through the family, the work mostly of women, by neighbours and friends, and through the various forms of self-help and mutual support groups through which the poor and the marginalized generally look after themselves. Situated neither as part of state activity, nor provided through the market, there is a vast network within civil society that embraces a wide range of human need and that attempts to meet the problems which people face.

Interestingly, this activity is rarely commented upon either in the media or in the academic press. There is little coverage, for example, of the sixty or more black educational projects currently active in the Leeds area which are attempting to provide a respectful and enriching education that black children so often find missing in state schools, or of the comparable Yemeni and Somali projects in Liverpool, Birmingham or Sheffield. Equally, little attention was drawn to the development of the network of well women clinics or rape crisis centres that developed from below from the 1970s onwards as women sought their own solutions to the problems of living in a patriarchal society. Popular welfare, whilst largely invisible from official gaze and outside commentary, nevertheless remains one of the most vital areas of collective and democratic activity. It encompasses all ages, from mother and toddler groups to old age pensioners' clubs. It exists in and through a huge variety of self-help groups, co-operatives, clubs, societies, organizations and associations, both formal and informal, in which millions of people are actively involved. Moreover, they do this not because they are paid or required to do so, but because they choose to.

In form and content this welfare is different from that associated with the state. In the first place it is popular. This is an obvious but not trivial point. Few parts of the welfare state could be said to have popular appeal. Perhaps the singular exception to this is the National Health Service, which in its origins stressed the importance of equality and the availability of free health care to all regardless of status or means. Its ability to tap the ideals of public service and the commitment of those who work for it has made it a focus of widespread popular, although still not unqualified, support. But few other parts of the welfare state can carry such support. Still less can they engage the active involvement of the mass of people, even, as when threatened, in their defence. This is particularly so for those parts of the welfare state that deal only or primarily with the poor. There has never, for example, been a grass-roots campaign for more social workers or more probation officers. On the contrary, to be associated with such services is to invite stigmatization.

Self-help on the contrary depends on popular support. It is by its very definition voluntary; no one is forced to take part in it. Although no statistics are available to gauge its size and extent, it is clear that millions of people of all ages freely devote their time and energy, and often their own resources, to keep organizations and networks going, sometimes in the face of considerable problems and challenges. Nothing sustains it other than the desire of those engaged in it to continue to be so. Examples of self-help of course come and go. Some have a permanence that has outlived generations; others are set up in response to an immediate need or situation and then disband. But what unites them is that they represent the free and autonomous self-organization of people for their own mutual benefit.

If self-help is, in the first place, popular, it is secondly rooted in popular life. It is not, as Jack Common described, 'the council school ... something clapped on us from above', but rather has grown out of the needs felt by poor and marginalized groups and communities and their own attempts to do something. As such it reflects people's own definition of their needs, as well as their preferred ways through which these needs might be met.

The ability to define a 'problem' is as important as the ability to say how it should be dealt with, and indeed the two are necessary parts of the same process. The power to define social problems has therefore been a crucial part of the politics of welfare, creating scope for a widening or narrowing of the range of what needs to be done. With respect to state welfare, it is usually others – policy-makers, officials or professionals – who define the problem and the ways it is to be dealt with. Frequently this has been done without consultation with those who are to be affected, whether they were the luckless tenants of the high-rise public housing developments of the 1960s or other victims of top-down urban redevelopment. Much of twentieth-century state welfare has been predicated, and indeed legitimated, on the fatuous assumption that 'ordinary people' are too stupid or disinterested to want to be involved in the planning of services to meet their needs. As we argue below, this has contributed to the profoundly anti-democratic character of state welfare regimes. The result can be at best a tremendous waste of energy and resources, as policies are developed which fail to take account of what people really need or want; at worst it is used to deny their reality and to impose on people policies which are inappropriate, counter-productive or oppressive.

If self-help reflects popular needs and allows people to define their own needs and wants, it also attempts to meet these needs in ways which reflect popular life and culture. It is by its very nature both relevant and accessible. When in 1844 chief factory inspector Leonard Horner reported to Parliament on the reasons for the miners' strike in County Durham, he noted that 'the colliers tend, in general, to prefer sending their children to the old kind of day schools kept by men of their own class, though the charges are higher than at the new schools under trained masters'; what was more, he added ominously, in place of the instruction that trained teachers could provide, 'the books they use are such as the parents choose to send' (quoted in Corrigan 1979: 35). This preference of the working class for working-class education provided by working-class people using books that they themselves chose to read meant that people's own lives were reflected in what (and how) they learned. In contrast, the gap between state schooling and the lived experience of working-class men and women has remained a constant source of alienation. The failure of state schools to speak to the experience of the poor or of ethnic minorities has been a factor both in patterns of inequality and in the continuing search for alternatives.

In the third and final place, popular welfare is pre-eminently collective. The values it supports and encourages are those of solidarity, democracy and mutual respect. This is in sharp contrast to state welfare, whose impact is to individualize, which has resisted democratic control, and which over much of its terrain does much to humiliate and degrade its recipients.

State welfare has in many ways been profoundly undemocratic. It is not simply that, as the welfare state has expanded, so the levers of political power and control have slipped ever further into the hidden recesses of an increasingly centralized state: government-appointed quangos now dominate much of state policy where once locally-elected Boards determined policy and practice in such areas as social security, health or education. It is also that, in the face of the popular pressure for democratic change, state welfare has become increasingly professionalized, entrusted to the hands of certificated (and largely middle-class) 'experts' who have ensured that ordinary people have been given little effective say. In some areas, such as medicine, this has long been the case: the history of the medical profession is in large part a history of the attempt by middle-class men, despite their historic incompetence and medical barbarism, to carve out a monopoly, and usurp the more general, unlicensed and unauthorized role of women as healers in their own communities (Ehrenreich and English 1979). Along with others who lay claim to professional monopolies and power, this has involved not merely legal restrictions on the ability or rights of others to practise a particular occupation. It has also involved the construction of a particular mystique, a vocabulary and a social practice which sets them apart as 'experts', and which leaves ordinary people feeling powerless to question or challenge their authority.

Self-help has little truck with 'experts', or at least the variety of expertise that has dominated state welfare provision and has constructed an elaborate system of planning, provision and delivery over which ordinary people are rarely consulted and from which they are, because of their lack of 'expertise' for the most part excluded. On the contrary, popular welfare has struggled to overcome the reign of experts: like the women's health movement, it seeks to challenge and demystify the jargon of consultants and doctors; to democratize access and decision-making; and to share the skills and knowledge of those involved.

What popular welfare also reveals in this process is the immense range and depth of skills, aptitudes and abilities that ordinary people possess. In countless examples it is the ingenuity of people often dismissed as having nothing to contribute that stands out: the ability to scrape together resources, to improvise, and to imagine. Some sense of this is offered by the architect Walter Segal, who was one of the key influences behind the Lewisham Self-Build Housing Association, through which local people on the local authority's housing waiting list in the late 1970s won the right to build their own homes. Colin Ward recalls how Segal was lyrical about their achievements and the ways in which the project changed their lives:

> It wasn't just a vindication of his building method and its relevance in a country with a need for cheap, quick yet durable housing, and with people in unsought idleness. It was a triumph for his belief that people could – if aided rather than pushed around – manage their own lives and shape their own environment. And instead of being dismayed at the 'countless small variations and innovations and additions' to the designs he had worked out with each individual family, he rejoiced that 'there is among the people that live in this country such a wealth of talent', and he found it unbelievable that this creativity would continue to be denied outlets.
>
> (Ward 1991: 100–1)

Organizations of popular welfare need to be seen as important political institutions, particularly for those who through their class, gender, 'race', age or ability are excluded from 'mainstream society' and its agencies. As countless local community groups show, they are frequently a testimony to the ways in which those who have been dismissed as uneducated and worthless can, given the opportunity, become centrally involved in managing complex organizations, demonstrating capacity, intelligence and sensitivities that have been systematically denied and thwarted. As such they constitute crucial prefigurative organizations which provide critical opportunities for democratic practice and debate. They are also, of course, often difficult places. Not immune from the culture and world around them, they can also be sites of conflict and division, intolerance and bigotry. It is no good pretending that building democratic institutions is always an easy and trouble-free process. But if the vision of socialism means anything it is the belief in the capacity of ordinary people to run their own lives.

It is in this collective experience that popular self-help is to be distinguished from bourgeois individualism. Although both may use the same term, they are worlds apart. Bourgeois self-help is rooted in a belief, to use Margaret Thatcher's infamous pronouncement, that 'there is no such thing as society, only individual men and women and families'; collective self-help, on the contrary, rests on a belief in the power of collective, social action. Their origins and consequences reflect fundamentally different political trajectories.

The politics of self-help

The relationship between popular welfare and state welfare is not confined to differences of style or approach. The existence of independent and autonomous working-class activity has always posed the greatest political challenge to those in power. This was evident in the birth of the trade union movement, as well as in the blossoming of political movements that greeted the Industrial Revolution, and in the responses developed to cope with the problems it created. Initially the threat was met with repression: workers' organization was outlawed; activists imprisoned or transported. But while repression remains a necessary response to the maintenance of the existing social order, in response to anti-poll tax riots or anti-road protesters, the suppression of popular struggle, and the popular welfare that has accompanied it, has called for tactics also to supplant, regulate, incorporate and defuse the challenge it poses. In this, the state and state 'welfare' has played a major part.

One of the most important, and enduring, examples of this was the state's response to working-class education. From the time of the Industrial Revolution onwards, a growing working class had recognized, in the words of the masthead of one of the most popular (and, after their suppression, illegal) of working-class newspapers, *The Poor Man's Guardian*, that 'Knowledge is Power'. The development of various forms of working-class self-education was to give focus to this pursuit, ranging from the miners' schools which Horner discovered, to night schools, Sunday schools, Chartist schools, reading rooms and other initiatives in which young and old, literate and illiterate came together to learn. Fiercely independent of the attempted influence of the established church, philanthropists, and later of the state, they were to embody the essential belief, as one advocate put it, that 'a people's education is safe only in a people's own hands' (quoted in

Hollis 1973: 65). They also gave the lie to the belief, subsequently enshrined in a number of accounts of the history of state welfare, that before state provision of education the mass of the people were uneducated and illiterate. On the contrary, as Engels noted in 1844:

> These different sections of working men ... have founded on their own hook numbers of schools and reading rooms for the advancement of education. Every socialist, and almost every Chartist institution, has such a place, and so too have many trades. Here the children receive a purely proletarian education, free from all the influences of the bourgeoisie; and, in the reading rooms, proletarian journals and books alone, or almost alone, are to be found. These arrangements are very dangerous to the bourgeoisie ... I have often heard working men, whose fustian jackets scarcely held together, speak upon geological, astronomical, and other subjects, with more knowledge than the most 'cultivated' bourgeois in Germany possess. ... And all are united on this point: that they, as working men, form a separate class, with separate interests and principles, and with a separate way of looking at things in contrast with that of all property-owners; and that in this class reposes the strength and the capacity of development of the nation.
>
> (Engels 1958 [1892]: 234–5)

Such developments did not long withstand the attention of Britain's ruling class, although perhaps the common disbelief in the capacity of ordinary people, combined with feuding amongst the different religious denominations about what sort of education should take its place was to delay decisive state action for a surprisingly long time. In 1854 *The Times* warned its readers of the dangers of delay:

> The education of the people has been constantly discussed for many years. ... Meanwhile the character and conduct of the people are constantly being formed under the influences of their surroundings. While we are disputing which ought to be the most beneficial system of education, we leave the great mass of the people to be influenced by the very worst possible teachers. ... In 1850 Harney's Red Republican has published in full 'The Communist Manifesto' supporting every revolutionary movement against the existing social and political order of things. ... The National Reform League is campaigning for the nationalisation of land, atheism is being actively propagated. ... Cheap publications containing the wildest and the most anarchical doctrines are scat-

tered, broadcast over the land. ... The middle classes may find it hard to believe in such atrocities. Unfortunately they know little of the working classes; only now and then, when some startling fact is brought before us, do we entertain even the suspicion that there is a society close to our own of which we are as completely ignorant as if it dwelt in another land, and spoke a different language, with which we never conversed, and in fact we never saw. ... Only in one way can this great danger, this great evil be counteracted. The religious sects must bury their differences. Let prudent spirit of conciliation enable the wise and the good to offer to the people a beneficial education in the place of this abominable teacher.

(quoted in Corrigan 1979: 31–2)

It was not, however, until 1870 that the Elementary Education Act was to establish for the first time a system of state schooling for the working class: a provision that was to be made compulsory just over a decade later. In so doing the state was to attempt to replace 'dangerous knowledge' with 'useful knowledge', and thus subvert the radical potential that working-class self-education threatened. In more telling ways, schooling was to take the place of education: the liveliness, vitality and thirst for education that had characterized working-class self-education was replaced by the numbing routine, boredom and monotony of an alien system that was to lead generations of working-class children to resist its imposition and leave at the earliest possible opportunity.

In addition to confusing working-class self-help with its bourgeois opposite, critics have also dismissed self-help as reactionary, diversionary, or at best a limited defence against a system which needs instead to be overthrown. This is to misunderstand the nature of political struggle. Self-help is certainly defensive; it is how individuals and communities protect themselves and attempt to meet unsatisfied needs. But this always takes place in a context – of who is being defended against and who is responsible for the need. In the process, self-help builds on, generates and sustains alternative explanations and visions, critiques of and challenges to the status quo, and a basis for its transformation. Richard Hoggart captures a sense of this in his reflections on the welfare state:

When I look back on my childhood in Hunslet, a working class district in Leeds, the aspects which have a special bearing on present changes are these. First, a quite deeply rooted sense that

we are at the thin end of society ... that we lived in the grimy
south of the town, on the wrong side of the river. On the other
side there was a rather shadowy impalpable 'them': local authorities, Rating officers, Public Assistance officers, Welfare officers ...
There was this initial imaginative divide between us. We knew in
our bones that this separation existed. ... As a kind of reaction to
this there was also a quite tight sense of being a local neighbour-
hood; a sense of belonging to an area and a group. Much of this
sense was defensive, obviously, but when you look at it closely,
you see that it was not merely defensive. What impresses, I think
more than anything, is the virtues it sustained. If you examine
some of its more obvious expressions such as the creation of co-
operatives and friendly societies; or if you think of the interweav-
ing of Christianity, socialism, a traditional 'peasant' community
sense, a defensiveness against the bosses, and see how all these
things came together in one texture, then you are struck by the
intricacy – the extraordinary depth, strength and charity – of that
texture.

(Hoggart 1960: 13)

It is this institutionalization of popular welfare within the culture of
poor communities that sustains it not only as a form of support and
defence against the outside world, but also as an implicit, if not
explicit, critique of the way that the outside world does things and
what it has to offer. The banner of the Nottinghamshire and
Derbyshire Coal Miners' Association depicting a widow who, when
faced with having to apply for Poor Law relief, announced that her
late husband's membership of the association and its benefit scheme
meant that 'she did not have to obey "the dictator" when he told her
to "sell off her furniture" '(Benson 1975: 403), symbolized more than
just the ability of trades unions and Friendly Societies to protect their
members; it also said something about the working-class view of the
state. Nurtured within its institutions of collective defence, this
suspicion of and hostility towards the state and the interests it
represented was, by the beginning of the twentieth century, to become
a major cause of political concern amongst the British ruling class, and
the attempt to overcome it a major objective of social reform.

As we noted at the beginning of this chapter the social reforms
introduced largely by a Liberal government before the First World
War that laid the framework of the twentieth-century welfare state
were not reforms demanded by the working class, and were indeed

undertaken against the critical hostility of many. As one contemporary supporter of reform observed:

> the present movement of social reform springs from above rather than below. The cry for an eight hours bill, for further factory legislation, for improvement of sanitation, for the readjustment of the incidence of taxation, or old age pensions, is less the spontaneous demand of the working classes than the tactical inducement of the political strategist.
>
> (Atherley-Jones 1893: 629)

As a political strategy from above, social reform was to attempt to overcome the political alienation and hostility of the mass of working-class people towards both capitalism and its state. Given a state whose welfare policy, until then, was enshrined in and largely limited to a deterrent and punitive Poor Law, such hostility was not surprising. But in a context of increasing political, and at times revolutionary, consciousness it was argued that something needed to be done, as Sidney Webb put it, 'to promote in every way the feeling that "the Government" is no entity outside of ourselves, but merely ourselves organised for collective purposes, regarding the State as a vast benefit society, of which the whole body of citizens are necessarily members' (Webb 1890: 104).

Over the following years social reformers were to press for a realignment of state policy that would offer a more benign and positive form of welfare to those who would now be regarded as citizens rather than outcasts. And in so doing, social reform would seek to replace working-class self-help as the principal means through which provision was made against the threats of sickness, unemployment or old age. Given the immense financial strain that prolonged unemployment and poverty imposed on working-class Friendly Societies, the offer of a state-subsidized old age pension was, in the view of the Ancient Order of Foresters, the second largest and one of the most 'respectable' of Friendly Societies, 'a very alluring bait to obtain the support of the friendly societies', but, he went on, 'concealed under the bait, to use an angler's illustration, is an insidious hook, which would drag us out of the waters of self-dependence and land us on the enervating bank of state control' (quoted in Chamberlain 1892: 607).

It was, however, not simply control of working-class self-help that was at stake. The project of state social reform was to 'seek to discern the real aspirations of the "dim inarticulate" multitude, and to guide and interpret these into safely effective political action' (Webb 1890:

120). 'Safe' political action in this context meant guiding the working class into a belief in and support for parliamentary reform, as opposed to extra-parliamentary struggle and change. To achieve this would require a repackaging of the state, so that it was no longer to be experienced simply as an alien and hostile institution, against which working-class self-help sought to defend itself, but as representing a 'national' interest and offering rights and benefits, at least to those whose political alienation threatened it most. In this project, social reform was to play a central part. It was, in the words of the German Emperor Bismarck, 'a duty of State-preserving policy, whose aim should be to cultivate the conception that the State is not merely a necessary but a beneficent institution' (quoted in Corrigan 1977: 386). The social reforms introduced earlier in Germany, in the face of perhaps the most revolutionary working-class movement in Europe, were held out as a shining example, and English social reformers flocked to study and learn from its experience. As one reported:

> The English progressive will be wise if, in this at any rate, he takes a leaf from the book of Bismarck, who dealt with heaviest blow against German socialism not by his laws of oppression ... but by that great system of State insurance which now safeguards the German worker at almost every point in his industrial career.
>
> (quoted in Gilbert 1966: 257)

A belief in the power and ability of the state to solve the problems of poverty and inequality within capitalism was a project which the co-operative movement had warned some sixty years earlier 'begins in delusion and ends in disappointment' (Youngjohns 1954: 32). As early as 1842, in debate with supporters of the Chartist movement, the founder of the Glasgow co-operative society, Alexander Campbell, spelled out his views of the limits and dangers of parliamentary democracy with a foresight that later working-class leaders would have done well to imitate:

> He was well aware that the Chartists supposed that if they had the Charter, then they would be able to send such parties to Parliament as would make those laws which were required for the good of the people. Now, he must submit that so long as class organisation existed, so long must class legislation exist ... that would be true equally under a monarchy, or a republic, so long as society was divided into classes. As a proof that a republican form of government was not of itself sufficient to remove the state of

anarchy, confusion, and want of employment among the poor, he might refer them to America, where they had had more than Chartist institutions for more than half a century, but where they had merely changed the form of government without changing the form of society.

(Quoted in Youngjohns 1954: 26)

At the beginning of the twentieth century the lure of social reform was, however, to prove very difficult to resist, although many remained suspicious of its motivation and intent. The dilemma of reformism that was subsequently to haunt working-class politics was that the state offered immediate and tangible benefits, in the form of old age pensions or insurance against sickness and unemployment, while the prospect of more fundamental change remained a more hazardous and distant project.

Although most remained sceptical of what the state had to offer, the dilemma of reformism was that few could easily reject its immediate benefits. Middle-class reformers were to exploit this dilemma, presenting state social reform as 'socialism' itself. Between themselves, of course, they continued to draw a distinction; as one put it, 'there are socialists and Socialists. ... The socialists with a big "S" have proved immensely serviceable to the more rational body of reformers by forcing inquiry upon sluggish minds' (Arnold 1888: 560). Or as another saw it:

If we are all socialists now, as is so often said, it is not because we have undergone any change of principles of social legislation, but only a public awakening to our social miseries. ... We are all socialists now, only in feeling as much interest in these grievances as the Socialists are in the habit of doing, but we have not departed from our old lines of social policy.

(Rae 1890: 439)

Indeed, although the introduction of National Insurance, old age pensions, and a host of other state-sponsored reforms before the First World War would vastly increase the role of the state, the fundamental lines of social policy – its power to distinguish between the deserving and the undeserving, to reinforce divisions and inequalities, and in general to support rather than challenge the operation of a capitalist market – would remain. This was a point not lost on many working-class activists. 'State socialism,' George Holyoake warned his members in the co-operative movement, 'means the promise of a dinner, and a bullet when you clamour for it' (Holyoake 1878: 510).

Conclusion

During the course of the twentieth century, popular politics have been directed towards a belief that state welfare could solve people's problems. The sense of purpose and agency in this is deliberate. Although it originated as a strategy from above, it was also to be taken on and pursued by leading sectors of the labour movement, partly through the trades unions but most notably through the Labour Party. The social democratic belief in the capacity for the progressive reform of capitalism, and the use of the state as a means to achieve this, reached its height in the welfare state that was created after 1945. In many respects, substantial and important gains were made for people's welfare. Benefits were extended; many experienced a reduction in the insecurities that characterized working-class life; access to an expanding range of education, housing and health services was widened. Yet these gains also came at a cost, and, as the experience of growing poverty and inequality and the retrenchment of the welfare state during the 1980s and 1990s has shown, they were to prove tenuous and relatively short-lived.

One of the significant costs of the expansion of state welfare was a loss of popular and democratic control and influence. Just as social democracy grew so democratic control receded. Local control over the social security system, exercised for some hundreds of years when only the wealthy exercised political rights, was gradually withdrawn into an increasingly centralized state bureaucracy; education committees supplanted local school boards, and have in turn been largely displaced through central government control; quangos and other appointed bodies now dominate public life and decision-making as the state has responded to popular participation in its institutions by drawing in the levers of power. With the expansion of the welfare state, the power of the welfare professions also grew immensely. Social workers, teachers, doctors, town planners and architects all 'knew best' what ordinary people needed. Few ever thought it necessary to ask them what they wanted. Indeed, as in social work, what clients said they wanted (such as respite from the pressures of childcare or money to buy food) was, in the jargon of the profession, simply a 'presenting problem' hiding more deep-rooted and much more important psychological problems beneath. For many, state welfare was and remains a deeply contradictory experience: providing for essential needs, but in ways which are often felt to be alien and oppressive, and over which they have little say and impact.

It is in this context that popular self-help has continued to form an important part of people's welfare. It is in itself not the solution to the problems of poverty and inequality that millions of people face. The fundamental problems of unemployment and insecurity, the gross inequalities of wealth and income, the lack of decent housing, health or education are not going to be overcome simply by people providing their own welfare, without a challenge to the forces and factors that create these problems in the first place. But such a challenge needs to learn from, to build upon and to nurture the visions and capabilities that it represents, without which a popular solution is impossible.

4 Class struggle and the origins of state welfare reform

John Charlton

Introduction

The decades leading up to the First World War have widely been recognised as the seed-bed of the modern welfare state. It is a judgement which can be sustained. The new Poor Law of 1834 was the first major excursion by the capitalist state into the area of social policy. Bureaucratic and coercive though it had been from its outset, its central objective continued to be the enforcement of *laissez-faire* economics; the exclusion of the state from the economic arena. Its contradictory core, however, could not for ever sustain its operation. Yet it was almost forty years before a cycle of state activity began.

Forster's Education Act, enforcing schooling on workers' children, was delivered in 1870, and by 1914 governments had performed a range of policy initiatives covering public health, working-class housing, the Poor Law, social insurance, industrial compensation, pensions for the elderly and, perhaps centrally, unemployment. The specific measures were largely drawn up following a series of intense inquiries and reports. Only the Poor Law Report of 1834 (see Chapter 2), and a few early inquiries into conditions in certain industries, bear comparison in their detail with these reports, but nothing earlier could compare with the flurry of activity in this period culminating in those which followed the 1906 general election.

While much investigation was unofficial, for example the work of Charles Booth and Seebohm Rowntree, by 1914 the state was quite clearly the major agent of investigation and interference in the lives of its citizens, and especially of the working-class section of the population (Langan and Schwarz 1985). We can better understand the scope of this activity if definition of what is included in state interest and intervention is drawn widely to include industrial relations and even, if more peripherally, such areas as working men's transportation.[1] It makes no sense to separate the 'coercive' state from the 'welfare' state or the 'facilitating' state, except for analytical purposes.

Nevertheless, even narrowly drawn to include only what is conventionally considered 'social welfare' the range of measures instituted by the Liberals, following their landslide victory in 1906, is impressive. Though often the specific steps taken were modest some important 'principles' were conceded or established. Three key areas were the subject of reform: unemployment, national insurance and health care. Labour Exchanges were established and, grudgingly, benefits were to be paid, notionally, at least, separating unemployment from moral torpor. Trade boards were founded to establish minimum standards for workers in certain occupations. Modest old age pensions were to be paid on the basis of contributions, as too were sickness benefits. Legislation was brought forward to permit the provision of school meals and milk and facilities were made available to standardize midwifery and children's medical treatment. Much of the legislative initiatives stemmed from the recommendations of the Majority and Minority Reports of the Poor Law Commission (1905–9). Its establishment was in itself a strong indicator of a sea-change in ruling-class thinking since its objectives breached traditional views on poverty and the poor (Bruce 1968).

Class conflict and the shift from a *laissez-faire* attitude

The dramatic shift of thinking by the ruling class from a rampant *laissez-faire* attitude to a position bordering on corporatism in such a short time-span was unrivalled historically. Some account of this shift in climate is necessary. Explanations, contemporary and subsequent, have been varied and contentious. That the debate took place at all suggests a considerable change in Britain's material circumstances. It is incontrovertible that in the second half of the nineteenth century Britain moved from a position of virtual world economic hegemony to one of fierce and violent competition creating a growing attitude of self-doubt among the leading opinion formers (Hobsbawm 1978, 1987).

Economic turbulence was much intensified by the onset of a cyclical world recession after 1873. Rationalization as one response to the economic downturn advanced the national over the regional and the general over the sectoral. Britain's became a truly national economy. Stresses and tensions were felt nationally. Technical and organizational innovation was a second response to crisis. Factors interacted to produce serious effects on the population. Craft skill was threatened and serially undermined. Few workers were insulated from periodic unemployment. Tens of thousands formed vast pools of short- and long-term unemployment. Tremendous strain was put upon the existing Poor Law in financing it and executing it. The debate on how to deal with changing circumstances raged within and without the ruling class. The outcome was an incremental shift in the state's engagement.

Explanation of this shift has been a busy terrain for historians and social scientists with a number of well-worked positions. First, it was argued, there was the well-honed sentiment of paternalism. Appalled by the realization of the plight of their fellow citizens, observed, it is true, across a vast gulf of incomprehension, significant numbers of ruling-class members set out from humanitarian motives to improve the lot of the poor. There is plenty of evidence to support this view. A generation of upper-class ladies visited the slums to dispense charity (see Mooney 1998). Upper-class chaps travelled to the East End of London to do service to the poor between Oxbridge and careers in the City, church or colonial service. Such activities can easily be seen as running in parallel with their perhaps more intrepid counterparts who journeyed to 'Darkest Africa' to take 'civilization' to the natives.

If the first impulse was sympathy and service, supported by an outpouring of Christian charity (Inglis 1963), fostered it must be said in some of the mid-Victorian public schools like Dr Arnold's Rugby, it was soon supplemented, though not necessarily replaced, by a harder-edged variety. This was not largely the dispensation of charity but social enquiry, precise and painstaking by the standards of the day. Whilst there was no particular reason why the former visitations should lead to a call for state intervention rather than private charity this was not true of the latter. Meticulous social enquiry would reveal a scale of problem surprising in its enormity. The most famous example of this was Charles Booth's reports. Booth, scion of a bourgeois Liverpool family, commenced his investigation into the situation of the London poor to prove strident socialists wrong. His first study, to do with poverty in East London (Booth 1889), found that 35 per cent, or 314,000 people, were 'poor', over 100,000 of whom suffered from acute 'distress'. His activity led him to devote the rest of his life to further investigation and pressure on the state to act. The problems were much too serious to leave to private initiative alone.

Also from within the ruling class came what may be called the instrumental view. For survival Britain needed to augment its Empire. The ruling class could supply administrators from within its own ranks. The public school system and Oxbridge would see to that. But it was necessary to win and hold territory. This required an army. The rulers could supply the officer corps, but not the rank and file soldiers. They would come from the working class. Hinted at for years, and apparently confirmed by reports on recruitment for the Boer War, was the fact that substantial parts of the working class were in a debilitated physical condition; in no fit state to fight. The state must act. Empire was at stake.

Imperialism also figured large in another strand of thought (Semmel 1960). Not only should soldiers be physically fit to fight, they should also want to fight. Moreover those fighting should be fighting with the consent of those at home in the factories, mines and railroads. A class wracked by poverty and humiliated by subservience could by no means be guaranteed either to fight or happily consent to massive expenditure on imperial projects. Again, the state must act to stave off revolt if not revolution. As early as 1885 Samuel Smith remarked in the *Contemporary Review*:

> I am deeply convinced that the time is approaching when this seething mass of human misery will shake the social fabric, unless we grapple more earnestly with it than we have done. ... The proletariat may strangle us unless we teach it the same virtues which have elevated the other classes of society.
>
> (Samuel Smith, cited in Perkin 1989: 54)

Each of the above explanations for the increased intervention of the state have some force. The intentions and impact of those engaged may be charted and assessed to a greater or lesser degree. It has been done exhaustively and it is not part of the argument of this chapter to cover that ground again. Our project is to consider the salience of class struggle in the changing situation. In fact, class division is at the heart of each of the arguments. That is, they all proceed from the recognition that the rewards dealt out in society are distributed unequally.

Poverty is certainly recognized as a serious outcome of inequality. Most protagonists of these positions would acknowledge the salience of class in their analysis and some would be conscious of the working classes, or even the working class singular, as a dynamic and threatening presence. Some positions veered towards seeing the working class as poor, passive victims, others towards a louring potentially violent presence. So, in a sense the latter could be seen as supporting a class struggle thesis of reform, though the argument is complex.

The important question is how far a class struggle thesis of social reform can be sustained. The argument has to operate on more than one level. First, and must obviously, did the ruling class react to upsurges in open class struggle by offering palliatives? Was there a direct link between, say, the revolt of the unskilled at the end of the 1880s and specific reforms? Evidence of this sort would be important but extraordinarily difficult to establish for this period.

Evidence that ruling classes operate so directly is available. In the Paris 1968 uprising, for example, the French government produced a hasty reform programme at the height of the struggle for the streets and factories. It was clearly true of Britain in the early to mid-1970s. The Wilberforce Report gave the miners almost everything they had demanded in 1972; the Social Contract delivered much of their agenda in 1974. However, both relied heavily upon the presence of an influential trade union leadership which could seek and receive offers and mediate between the state and the class. In the late nineteenth century no such effective agency existed. Yet in August of 1889 a rudimentary process of this kind was initiated by Cardinal Manning to bring about the ending of the Great Dock Strike and strike wave of that summer (Charlton 1999). It may have hinted at future possibilities of arbitration but its objectives were quite limited and cannot be directly linked to the growth of state intervention. We would, therefore, by definition be looking for something much less direct.

A second inflection of the argument would be to look for a delayed reaction to big events. Here the ruling class might respond by engaging in a debate within its ranks after excitement had subsided. In some circumstances the outcome might be a reform or a series of reforms. On the other hand it might lead to a retaliatory employers' offensive. This may also be seen in the early 1890s where employer obduracy actually grew after the strike wave. Delayed action might take place a few months or a year after an event or even a decade or more afterwards to the point where no connection is obvious. Yet, it might be there in the sense that a resonance of struggle planted in the ruling-class consciousness might take considerable time to work itself through in thought and practice. Career trajectory might be an important variable. An example may illuminate this point. The best middle-class eyewitness account of the strike events of 1889 was that of Llewellyn Smith, who was at that time a minor civil servant. As Sir Hubert Llewellyn Smith he was Permanent Secretary at the Board of Trade from 1907–19 and a major planner of the new unemployment insurance scheme in 1907. It is possible that his awareness of potential either took two decades to mature or that he had not previously been in a position to effect in practice long-held views.

A yet third inflection could be reform coming after a period of relatively minor working-class actions. In such a case where these actions took place, perhaps on a rising curve, reformist elements within the ruling class might use such manifestations to warn the ruling class at large of trends which might best be contained by reforming responses. Finally, a fourth inflection could be a spate of reform apparently responding to no obvious working-class actions. Would such a situation mean that the class struggle interpretation lost all force? I do not believe so, but it might require a qualitatively different understanding of the class struggle terminology. A spate of reform might derive from a sense in the ruling class of a growing working-class presence not necessarily related to specific militant manifestations of action, but in perceptions of its size, growth, population concentration, the existence of working-class organization like trades unions, co-operatives, Friendly Societies, and of mass leisure activities.

The working-class presence in late Victorian Britain

There is much to suggest that the last quarter of the nineteenth century and the period up to the outbreak of the First World War was just such a period. The population was approximately 22 million in 1851. By 1901 it was over 38 million. The working-class sector had grown much faster than that of other classes. There were 65 per cent more miners, 62 per cent more transport workers, 66 per cent more metalworkers, 67 per cent more building workers, and these workers were increasingly living in large urban concentrations. Workers' districts had emerged (Charlton 1992; Hobsbawm 1984) in the big cities: Attercliffe, Tinsley, and Hillsborough in Sheffield; Gorton, Openshaw and Trafford Park in Manchester; Hunslet, Holbeck and Armley in Leeds; Heaton, Walker, Elswick and Scotswood in Newcastle; Govan, Partick and Clydebank on Clydeside and Smethwick, Saltley and Aston in Birmingham. Increasingly, gentlemen attended these areas only for business or crossed them on the way to business. Socially integrated housing was rapidly declining and workers' housing was becoming physically recognizable. Serried ranks of small regular streets crossed the factory districts. Workers congregated and socialized in the same places: pubs, music halls, football matches and day trips to Blackpool, Porthcawl, Whitley Bay and Bridlington. They had their own churches. Dialect and accent once more widely shared became the workers' badge. The sense of social segregation was almost absolute.

All this, though, describes the working class as a presence but a relatively passive one. That was telling enough for the middle-class observer. But what was worse was its active face. Here there were different experiences. There was the activity of the large crowd. At 'the match', by the 1890s, the crowds were measured in tens of thousands. Occasionally they rioted. In summer holiday weeks the railway stations were crowded with workers' families taking day trips. In the evenings and at weekends the streets were teaming with people. More ominously, in the mid-1880s there was a series of mass demonstrations, staged largely in London, protesting against unemployment, the persecution of the Irish and restrictions on free speech. All excited much comment in the press from long analytical articles in the dailies to lurid cartoons in weekly magazines. Few expressed the sense of 'presence' better than C. F. G. Mastermann, the Liberal philosopher-politician. In 1909, he wrote,

> You may see it in the dim morning of every London day, struggling from the outskirts of the city in to tramcars and trains which are dragging it to its centres of labour: numberless shabby figures hurrying over the bridges or pouring out of the exits of the central railway stations. You may discern in places the very pavements torn apart, and tunnels burrowed in the bowels of the earth, so that the astonished visitor from afar beholds a perpetual stream of people emerging from the middle of the street, seemingly manufactured in some laboratory below. It flows ... like a liquid unprecipitated ... but at any moment an unexpected incident may change the liquid from clear to cloudy, or reveal ... the debris and turgid elements ... men's voices are raised in altercation, an itinerant agitator demands work for all. ... The multitude of the unimportant gather together having hopes. With incredible rapidity appear among them the criminal, the loafer, the enthusiast. ... There is a note of menace in it ... the evidence of possibilities of violence in its waywardness, its caprice, its always incalculable mettle and temper ... the smile may turn into fierce snarl or savagery. ... Humanity has become the Mob.
>
> (Mastermann 1960: 23)

Observations such as this one are a confirmation of the growing awareness of the working-class presence with its unease. Yet in its way it is naïve, unfocused and thus fairly innocuous. It could prepare its audience equally for a bout of reform as for brutal confrontation. Not so the growing virulence directed at so-called 'aliens'. One commentator unsubtly linked labour militants and 'aliens' at the height of New Union agitation. 'We must prevent them growing into a body at once more noxious and more disliked than they already are. Mr Burns and Mr Tillett and Mr Mann could raise a Judenherze tomorrow if they like to do. It is for the prudent statesman to cut away the ground from under their feet' (Fishman 1975: 61). W. H. Wilkins accused the Jews of importing the principles of 'secret socialistic or foreign revolutionary societies' (Fishman 1975: 77). During the 1890s and into the new century the cry for restriction of aliens increased. They were linked with unemployment, poor housing conditions and disease. Agitation moved from the margins to the political centre becoming part of Tory Party policy which in 1905 culminated in the restrictive Aliens Act.

It would be wise, too, to embrace ruling-class knowledge of the international situation. It was a long attested feature of British society to see foreigners as heated revolutionaries and republicans alongside a calmer, passive, patriotic Britisher. Such an engrained view might have encouraged complacency among the rulers but such events as the Paris Commune, the rise of the Social-Democratic Party (SPD) in Germany, the serial violence of labour struggles in the United States[2] and the 1905 revolution in Russia, did not go unnoticed in Britain. The future Tory leader, Arthur Balfour, described the Liberal election victory in 1906 as 'The faint echo of the same movement which has produced massacres in St Petersburg, riots in Vienna and socialist processions in Berlin'. As well, there were always upheavals in Ireland to excite prejudice and produce fear.

When this experience is seen next to an undoubted quickening of industrial activity it must have appeared even more menacing for that also threatened the pockets of the rulers. It is sometimes thought that between the demise of the Chartists and the late 1880s the working class was marked by its passivity. It is true that there were few political mass movements. There was a short-lived, yet effective movement around the suffrage in 1866–67 and a few smaller political upsurges. On the other hand, industrial struggle never disappeared. Every year there were numerous strikes in industries up and down the country (Charlton 1992). Textiles and coal mining were especially strike-prone industries, but were by no means the only ones. Strikes could be long lasting, marked by bitterness and violence. Most strikes were of craft workers and coal miners. This fact dispels, at least partly, the view that skilled workers were passively consenting to class relations in the capitalist society. Rather, the situation was quite a complex one. On the one hand they were certainly sectional in their approach to the work situation. Some of this may have come out in their communities too. However they would fight with determination for their status. At a rank and file level they could by no means be seen as pushovers ready to co-operate. Of course they *had* to fight for their positions because the employers were far from compliant themselves. Despite the statistical evidence that employers remained obdurate and determined to assert their authority at all costs, there was a growing and uneasy recognition among the employing class that confrontation was not a productive means of solving disputes. In 1885, for example, a prestigious conference was held in London to discuss remuneration. Among its participants were Sir Thomas Brassey (son of the great railway contractor), the Earl of Dalhousie, A. J. Balfour (the future Tory prime minister), R. Giffen (of the Board of Trade), David Dale (the Darlington ironmaster), and several MPs and trade unionists. Following this was the establishment in 1893 of a Labour Department at the Board of Trade to record and monitor disputes. Its first secretary was John Burnett, a former leader of the Engineers Union. His early reports were definitely conciliatory in tone.

The situation was compounded in the late 1880s when the unskilled mass upsurge occurred. This upsurge came from groups of workers who had been almost completely disregarded. They had had virtually no success in organizing and, with a few small exceptions, were unrepresented by national or even local organizations. From the summer of 1887 when the Northumberland miners struck for twelve weeks and paraded along village lanes, to the Bolton engineers that autumn, to the match girls in the summer of 1888, the scene was set for the great mass activity of 1889.

For a period, from spring 1889 to spring 1891 and peaking in August, the working class demonstrated a sort of 'runaway consciousness'. Although there were precedents – the Beckton mass recruitment and the Great Dock Strike have been claimed as the midwife of new unionism. But it is not necessary to separate them nor is it really possible. They overlapped in time – March to September 1889. They overlapped in place – the strike began at the West India Dock just a mile or so from Beckton. Family members took part in both. Certainly neighbours must have done. Their leaders interlocked – Thorne, Burns, Tillett, Champion, Mann. Eleanor Marx and Annie Besant were involved with many disputes. Most had worked together as socialist agitators for years. Many had had their heads bashed by policemen's truncheons. Their papers reported the progress of the movement and circulated in the community.

Running in parallel with the dock strike, and lasting until the end of September 1889, was a strike of Jewish tailoring workers. Its centre was Stepney, the district adjacent, and to the west, of Canning Town in London. It was a big and militant strike of over 6,000 workers with 120 workshops reported idle. Like so many of the strikes in this period it was led by members of the Social Democratic Federation (SDF) who had been agitating among the tailors since 1885. The tailors had been very active in the movement against unemployment.

As significant as the tailors' strike, but never referred to in detail, was a proliferation of disputes in the second half of August and the beginning of September 1889. In London, within a rough triangle between the City, Kings Cross and Blackwall, points approximately five miles apart, there were over fifty strikes in industries other than the docks. Outside that triangle in south and west London there were at least a further sixteen strikes. There was also a report of a rent strike on Commercial Road. 'As we are on strike landlords need not call', warned a banner over Hungerford Street with the accompanying rhyme:

> Our husbands are on strike; for the wives it is not honey
> And we all think it is not right to pay the landlord money.
> Everyone is on strike; so landlords do not be offended.
> The rent that's due we'll pay when the strike is ended.
> (*Newcastle Daily Chronicle* 1889)

It was obvious that London was in ferment. Contemporaries knew it. *The Evening News and Post* proclaimed that 'The proverbial small spark has kindled a great fire which threatens to envelop the whole metropolis' (27 August 1889). *The East London Advertiser* warned that 'strike operations [had] such general proportions as to make the rising a war between capitals and labour' (31 August 1889). Meanwhile, the main editorial of *The East London News* was headlined 'STRIKE FEVER' and argued that:

> the present week might not inaptly be called the week of strikes – coal men, match girls, parcels postmen, carmen, rag, bone and paper porters and pickers and the employees in jam, biscuit, rope, iron, screw, clothing and railway works have found some grievance, real and imaginary, and have followed the infectious example of coming out on strike.
> (7 September 1889)

Further afield, the *Newcastle Daily Courant* told its readers that 'all kinds of workmen, far removed from the docks are joining the movement' (27 August 1889). And the Bristol paper, *The Western Daily Press*, stated that 'the great strike of dock labourers has reached enormous dimensions. The infection has spread to other classes of labouring men and the result is that London is threatened with a state of siege as if a hostile fleet held the entrance to the Thames' (28 August 1889).

Following Beckton, the union drive ran through most of London's gas works in the summer and autumn of 1889, though with not the same success. Other industries in east London were also affected, including the rubber industry of Silvertown, to the east of West Ham, where Eleanor Marx was active in the autumn. On 19 November 1889, it was reported in the *East End News* that 'Some two hundred women marched up with the men to take part in a demonstration at Victoria Park. This marks a new and important feature in the history of trades unionism – the union of women with men for common good. Silvertown is so remote that it has escaped general attention. Yet here some three thousand persons have been out on strike for nearly ten weeks, the women having struck for the sake of their male comrades'.

The Silvertown dispute was a direct spin-off from the Dock Strike and the action of the gas stokers. So too was the battle for unionization at the South Metropolitan Gas Company that autumn. As both disputes broke out dockers and gas workers rallied round. The demonstrations and picket lines were supported, donations were given and collections taken throughout the East End and further afield. Both were long and bitter struggles and both ended in defeat as employers regained their footing after the heady days of August and September. The manner of the ending of the Dock Strike, the continuing battles on the docks and the closing down of the mass movement took a great toll on attempts to unionize in the immediate period which followed, especially in London. Beyond London the results were patchy, but with some successes.

The organizing union drive in the gas industry spread far and wide: including Cardiff, Wolverhampton, Sheffield, Manchester, Halifax, Hull, Tyneside and, most spectacularly, Leeds. In the winter of 1889–90 Leeds gas workers joined up to the union en masse and obtained the eight-hour day. The leaders of the municipal undertaking conceded to the workers' demands, but had a concealed plan to reinstate the twelve-hour day and smash the union in the summer slack period. In June 1890 they tried to import hundreds of blacklegs under the protection of the police and soldiers. Some sense of the workers' strength is given by the attendance of over 6,000 people on Leeds' first May Day march, including nearly 1,000 gas workers, hundreds of builders' labourers who had formed a new union in the previous summer, and a large contingent of tailoring workers who had struck successfully in the autumn of 1888.

When the council gas committee announced its 'new' arrangements a group of workers immediately struck and were followed two days later by almost the entire gas works' labour force. The blacklegs who had arrived by rail were harassed by crowds of Leeds workers, estimated to be up to 30,000 strong, slugging it out with police in the streets. Those blacklegs who did not leave town were kept under guard in the Town Hall. Finally, they were marched out towards the gas works, escorted by a large force of police, foot soldiers and carabineers. A journalist reported the scene as they approached the railway bridges by the gas works:

> The bridges were crowded with men, who had stormed Holbeck station, made their way down the line and taken possession of them; and there they massed piles of missiles. In addition, the roofs of the buildings on either side of the road were covered with men who had also provided themselves with ammunition ... the advanced guard was allowed to get under the bridges almost in safety. The victims the stone throwers wanted were the 'knobsticks'. ... As they came within range, the fire was directed with terrific force on them, all who followed. The scene that ensued SIMPLY DEFIES DESCRIPTION, bricks, stones, 'clinkers', iron belts, sticks, etc., were hurled into the air to fall with SICKENING THUDS AND CRASHES upon and amongst the blacklegs and their escorts.
>
> (Cited in Hendrick 1974: 24)

The scabs retreated. The council caved in. The union won.

Elsewhere, seamen flocked to their new union and in Southampton, Plymouth, Cardiff, Liverpool, Hull, Glasgow, Dundee and Dublin new dock worker unions rapidly emerged or slightly older ones grew in size. New unionism was particularly strong in Bristol. The *Western Daily Press* reported long and bitter strikes among Somerset Colliers at Radstock and Clandown. As one worker reminisced:

> The first strike occurred at Lysaght's Galvanised Iron Works and this was followed in varying succession by Tinn's Galvanised Iron Workers, the Gas Workers, Dockers, Stay Makers, Cotton

Operatives, Brush Makers, Hatters, Oil and Colour Workers, Pipe Makers, Coal Carriers, Scavengers, Box Makers, Cigar Makers, Tramways Men, Hauliers, Blue Factory Workers, Animal Charcoal Workers, etc. etc.

(*Bristol Labour Weekly*, June 1929)

In the north-east of England the new mood preceded the upsurge in London. In July 1889, Northumberland miners protested against further grants to the royal family and followed with a demand for a 5 per cent pay increase. Durham miners demanded a 10 per cent increase and an end to the sliding scale. Durham engine workers demanded a 20 per cent increase and Cleveland blast-furnace workers 4 per cent. On 3 August in Sunderland the newly-formed sailors' and firemen's union claimed recruitment of 60,000 in one year with branches in forty-seven ports. Middlesborough dockers launched a union on 9 August and on 13 August Gateshead chain-makers proclaimed their support for all strikers. On 19 August Consett coke-men claimed 1,000 new members within the previous two weeks and the Newcastle-based National Labour Federation announced twenty new branches and 'massive recruitment'.

By the end of August, several factories in Birmingham were contributing to the London dockers' strike fund and 'a procession of trade unionists went through the streets with collecting sheets on handcarts. A large sum was collected and a proposal made to call a Birmingham General Strike!' (*Manchester Guardian*, 1889). And among craft unionists in Lancashire, cotton workers registered the highest number of strikes in any industry. There were over 230 recorded in that year. Over twenty-five strikes are detailed in *The Cotton Factory Times* for the months of July, August and September in Burnley, Oldham, Bolton, Haslinden, Preston, Great Harwood, Failsworth, Bury, Rawtenstall, Blackburn, Bury, Chorley, Darwen, Royton and Earby. Some of the strikes involved thousands of workers, most hundreds, and they included weavers and spinners, the skilled and unskilled, men, women and children. The stated causes were wide-ranging: underpayment of agreed prices, pay cuts, working hours, heavy-handed supervision, victimization. *The Cotton Factory Times*, very much a tool of the union bureaucracy, was not warmly disposed to strikers. It was all too ready to spot the work of 'rowdy youths of 16–20' (27 September) and found 'it pleasing to say they have all gone back' (6 September), however, it did communicate a sense of unrest, 'strikes of weavers in Burnley are recently very common' (30 August).

There were also union drives among the unskilled in Dundee, Aberdeen and in several places in West Yorkshire. One of the most notable strikes was one at Manningham Mills in Bradford between December 1890 and April 1891. Over 5,000 workers struck – the majority of them women – in an attempt to resist wage cuts. It was a mass strike, with thousands of workers repeatedly in action during the five months and supported on the streets by other Bradford workers. The strikers fought the police for the right to march and hold meetings after the Mayor and Town Clerk banned them from both indoor and outdoor council-owned venues. The strike ended in defeat, however.

The new movement made itself felt on the streets too. On 4 May 1890 the first May Day demonstration took place in London. Engels wrote for a German workers' paper:

> [O]n May 4th, 1890 the English proletariat, rousing itself from forty years of hibernation, rejoined the movement of its class. ... Surrounding the seven platforms of the Central Committee were dense crowds as far as the eye could see, marching up with music and banners, over a hundred thousand in the procession, reinforced by almost as many who had come individually; everywhere harmony and enthusiasm, and yet order and organisation.
>
> (Engels 1962 [1892]: 32)

The strike wave itself was characterized by some very distinctive features. It was unambiguously an upsurge of the unskilled, though many groups of skilled workers were infected, making their own demands. It brought forward a central demand for the eight-hour day, though not necessarily in each separate dispute. It was very militant, each dispute involving usually thousands of workers and more often than not having the financial and often the physical backing of other workers in the town or area. There was often a complete lack of regard for the police, the soldiers and any other authority figures who stood in the movement's way. Its all-embracing character drove straight in to the Trades Union Congress (TUC), shaking up the sectional attitudes of the leaderships of the craft unions. It provoked the employing class into a vicious determination to destroy what they saw as the desire 'to confiscate capital'. Finally, most of the disputes were led by men, and some women, from both inside and outside the industries, who were proud to declare themselves socialists. It was truly a mass movement at once spontaneous, unexpected, uneven, spirited, inventive and subject to sudden changes of mood.

For Engels, 'New Unionism' was about more than establishing trade unions for unskilled workers. In 1892 he wrote:

> The new unions were founded at a time when the faith in the eternity of the wages system was severely shaken; their founders and promoters were Socialists either consciously or by feeling; the masses whose adhesion gave them strength, were rough, neglected, looked down upon by the working class aristocracy; but they had this immense advantage, that their minds were virgin soil, entirely free from the inherited 'respectable' bourgeois prejudices which hampered the brains of the better situated 'old' unionists. And thus we see now these new Unions taking the lead of the working class movement generally, and more and more taking in tow the rich and proud 'old' Unions.
>
> (Engels 1962 [1892]: 32)

What Engels had clearly observed in the events of 1888 to 1891 was the emergence of a new mass movement of workers coming together as a class, spearheaded by the 'rough' and 'neglected', pulling the more conservative elements behind them in a challenge to the 'eternity of the wages system'.

The employers' counter-assault on the unions resulted in workers' resistance becoming localized and fragmented. Victories were hard fought and infrequent. Success was often temporary. The few victories that were achieved do not seem to have inspired others to follow. Defeats were much more frequent and no doubt contributed to low morale among workers. Within three years there were almost no victories on the industrial front. The employers' offensive was a savage counter-attack. For the bosses ideas clarified quickly. A markedly harder set of attitudes became respectable in ruling circles. Even craft trades unions, which had been tolerated for twenty years, were now seen as the class enemy. Tillett's new union was quite beyond the pale:

> [The union] cares not whether men are ill or well paid; it is ever ready with a fresh demand. Concession does but whet its appetite; it claims for labour the whole of the profits made by labour and capital combined; it aims to be the absolute dictator of the conditions of toil; to say who shall work and what he shall receive. ... The principle which underlies the militant union is the principle of socialism ... it desires to confiscate capital. Something needed to be done.
>
> (Briggs and Saville 1960: 322)

The Times led the charge. As early as Christmas Eve 1889 it was advocating organized scab labour:

> Why should they [free labour or scabs] suffer themselves to be intimidated by a set of loud-voiced bullies, whose skins, we venture to say, are quite as tender as those of the honest men they coerce? The difference lies, we believe, in discipline and organisation. The bullies organise themselves, having nothing else to do, while the workers feel themselves isolated and undisciplined. Surely there is a function here for employers to discharge. They ought to take the lead in organising, disciplining, and encouraging men who wish to work. If picketing is legal ... then so it must be legal to picket the pickets.
>
> (quoted in Briggs and Saville 1960: 323)

In the early part of the Dock Strike the balance of opinion had been for the dock workers. But a combination of the large meetings and processions, the mass pickets, the workers unwillingness to accept the bosses' first offer, possibly the General Strike call (even though it was revoked), and the large donation from Australian workers, meant that opinion shifted to outright hostility. The proprietors of the South West Metropolitan Gas Company's militantly successful stand against Will Thorne's new union in December was acclaimed.

During the decade of the 1890s, the police and army would be further encouraged to take a more pro-active and often violent role. Striking workers could be shot, as indeed miners were at Featherstone in 1893. Employers were encouraged into vigorous resistance of union demands. Scab labour was actively organized and financed. In 1893, 50,000 cotton workers were locked out for ten weeks and returned to a 5 per cent reduction in wages. The engineers were locked out in 1894 and suffered a severe set-back as a result. The judiciary was encouraged to revise its interpretation of the unions' legal rights. This culminated in the Taff Vale case in 1901 in which the Amalgamated Society of Railway Servants and its moderate leadership was held responsible for damages arising from a strike.

Violent aggression towards the organized labour movement was not the only response from within middle-class circles. There were those who drew different conclusions from the events of 1889. A German observer, writing only three years later, marvelled at a movement 'originating not among the skilled and organised labourers, but among that hopeless "Reserve Army of Industry" into whose ranks drift all those who have nothing to offer but the mere strength of their arms'

(Schulze-Gaevernitz 1893: 155). He was astonished at 'the solidarity of the working classes and the force of public opinion', and attributed much of the success to the 'good sense' of the English workman, but more significantly to the active intervention of enlightened middle-class people in the cause of social peace. It was this kind of thinking which was important in the shift of the ruling class towards greater state intervention in social policy. In the guise of Fabianism this element was to have an enormous formative influence on the future Independent Labour Party and the Labour Party.

It is important to emphasize one other point about the attitude of the ruling class; one which unites almost all shades of opinion, from the most conservative to the most liberal. That is, of the necessity to preserve existing class relations. The left-leaning liberal wanted to maintain compliance, containment and discipline among working people. He might have been appalled at the shootings at Featherstone in 1893, but he did not raise an eyebrow at the steady augmentation of the state power in the form of increased police numbers in the second half of the nineteenth century. From 1858 to 1918 the number of officers grew from 18,000 to 56,000 (Farrell 1992). Critical though their role might be at moments of conflict, equally important was their ongoing presence on the streets dealing constantly with petty resistance to law and received morals.

Far from protesting against this situation, it was the liberal advocates of increased state involvement who were responsible for at least a part of the growing army of officials who circumscribed the lives of working-class people and their communities. Social workers, truancy officers, teachers, doctors and other health professionals gave the welfare agenda its particular stamp on the ground. They tended to operate within a set of dominant assumptions regarding class, nation and family and made open judgements about who was deserving of support. Such views reflected a predominant conception of a large section of the working class as feckless, drunken, profligate of its, admittedly, meagre resources and lacking in moral fibre. It required the vigilance and intervention of the medical and social work professions who staked out their claims, as experts, to determine working-class standards of family life (see Ross 1986; Lavalette 1994).

Sentiments such as these pervaded even the period's most popular measure, the granting of old age pensions. These modest payments were available to all who

> had not been imprisoned for any offence, including drunkenness
> ... were not aliens or wives of aliens, and could satisfy the pension

authority that they had not been guilty of 'habitual failure to work according to his ability, opportunity or need, for his own maintenance and that of his legal relatives'.

(Thane 1982: 83)

Middle-class moral intervention was particularly acute in the education of working-class children. From the first compulsory schooling in 1870, there was a strong emphasis on socialization as much as education. Always implicit were extremely limited educational aims hardly extending beyond the three Rs. Although a very narrow avenue might exist for the very brightest working-class children through scholarship, the overall drive was to inculcate a system of values stressing subordination and acceptance within a framework of retributive Christianity and love of Crown and Empire (see Davin 1996).

Conclusion

In this chapter evidence has been surveyed indicating that the ruling class recognized the increasingly active presence of a working class. Accordingly, they sought to contain the phenomenon by introducing elements of social welfare reform in the decades preceding the First World War, intensifying the project in the final decade before 1914. It was not a magnanimous gesture informed as it was by minimalism and restriction. Rather, it was a series of gestures aimed largely at reshaping the working class to the perceived requirements of the capitalist economy.

Towards the end of the nineteenth century, the working class was bigger, concentrated in proletarian districts, working in larger work spaces and possessed of more coherent organizations. Its activity from the mid-1880s to the early 1890s was widespread and intense. It provoked a considerable response from the state: violent, restrictive, interventionist and conciliatory. All these elements were to remain part of ruling-class strategy. Just before the Great War there was an even greater upsurge of militant working-class activity but the die had already been cast. The ruling class had lumbered into a rolling state intervention policy which was to be intensified by the requirements of the warfare state between 1914 and 1918. The powerful relationship between class presence and class struggle and the thrust towards a welfare state is palpable, reflecting interactions between rulers and workers which were to have strong policy and legislative outcomes.

Notes

1   The Cheap Trains Act 1883 was aimed at getting working men expeditiously to the work place, as much an example of state intervention in the interests of a flexible labour market than an act of benevolence to workers.

2   In 1886, for example, the right-wing press commended the signs of firmness across the Atlantic where six framed Anarchists were about to be executed in Chicago. This followed the previous year's Chicago May Day demonstration in Haymarket Square in which a bomb had been thrown by an *agent provocateur* after the rally had ended. The indicted men had not even been present when the bomb exploded. There was also praise in the press for Bismarck who had brought in anti-socialist laws in Germany in the 1880s in an attempt to crush the growing influence of the Social Democrats.

5 'The Clyde Rent War!'

The Clydebank Rent Strike of the 1920s

Seán Damer

Introduction

It hardly needs mentioning that the Glasgow Rent Strike of 1915 was a major event in the stormy days of the 'Red Clyde' which lasted from 1914 to 1922. It is discussed in a plethora of memoirs of the period (Crawfurd n.d.; Milton 1973; Gallagher 1978; McShane and Smith 1978) and has been the topic of much analysis, both academic and political (cf., Damer 1980; Englander 1983; McLean 1983; Melling 1983; Kenefick and McIvor 1996). Yet the interpretation of the Rent Strike is a matter of controversy between various commentators, for example the historian Joseph Melling and sociologists Manuel Castells and Peter Saunders who wish to depoliticize the events, and those such as myself who wish to interpret it from a Marxist point of view.

Melling, Castells and Saunders argue that the 1915 Rent Strike – and similar struggles elsewhere – is an event which should be detached from the issue of class struggle. They maintain that such struggles are *not* part of the working-class struggle against capitalism because they do not challenge the fundamental relationship between the bourgeoisie and the proletariat: the ownership of the means of production. They believe that these struggles are merely about 'consumption', or how large a slice of cake the working class can win from the state. To the contrary, I would argue that rent strikes, like the one of 1915, are *essential* aspects of the class struggle. The working class has to struggle where it stands and to fight oppression in whatever form it appears. Such struggles have to be theorized as part of a social totality, and so the divorce of the economic and political spheres, characteristic of Castells', Melling's and Saunders' theses, is totally illegitimate. Finally, in interpreting the events involved in such struggles, we have to analyse what the workers themselves claimed they were doing.

The main differences of opinion were aired as long ago as 1980 in articles by Melling and myself (see Melling 1980), while the former elaborated his position in a book published subsequently (Melling 1983). Castells added his view in the same year, while Saunders' contribution came a little earlier (Saunders 1981). Melling's position is that the 1915 Rent Strike was *not* a form of class struggle:

> There arose a mass resistance to rent rises and landlordism which possessed its own dynamic and significance autonomous from the socialist critique of capitalism, or even the Labour campaign for municipal housing.
>
> (Melling 1983: 114)

Castells reaches the same conclusion when he writes that:

> both from the point of view of the movement and from the point of view of its political effects, the Rent Strike appears as an episode of the class struggle. Yet the absence of any direct confrontation with the dominant factions of the capital, the deviation of the demands towards the request for state intervention, and the actual support of the capitalists for the new housing policies, clearly challenge any interpretation of the Glasgow Rent Strike as an anti-capitalist movement.
>
> (Castells 1983: 36–7)

After reviewing the original data gathered by both Melling and myself, Castells argues that the Rent Strike was in fact an 'urban social movement' whose struggles were confined to the 'sphere of consumption'. Saunders argues that the 'social investment' functions of the state have been removed from the local level to the national level, that is, struggles over basic economic strategies occur only at the level of the state. In other words, basic class struggles are now removed from – are distinct from – the arena of local struggles. Such struggles, in Saunders' account, are only about consumption:

> Urban struggles are constituted in the sphere of consumption on the basis of specific sectoral interests which may or may not coincide with class alignments. They are neither one aspect of class struggle, nor a different type of class struggle. They are, rather, a specific type of political struggle *distinct* from political struggles grounded in class interests and class antagonisms.
>
> (Saunders 1981: 275, my italic)

Saunders, then, is in the same camp as Castells and Melling. But his position leads to thoroughly pessimistic conclusions about the potential for labour gains at the level of the local state, and for socialist organization: 'To the extent that local government powers are limited to the sphere of social consumption ... such municipal victories will not necessarily undermine or affect key economic policies' (ibid.: 265). And he goes on to say that: 'It also means that those whose primary concern lies in furthering the conditions for the development of socialism will derive little return from either analysis of or activity in urban politics' (ibid.: 276).

Each one of these positions seems to me absurd. I would argue that both Melling's data and my own show unequivocally that the Glasgow Rent Strike was grounded in a socialist, working-class culture unique to that city, whose origins and attributes I have described elsewhere (Damer 1990), and was led by a talented cadre, the majority of whom were members of the Independent Labour Party (ILP), *the* working-class party in Glasgow at the time. If that does not constitute a working-class struggle, it is hard to see what would. If, as Melling has argued, the 1915 Glasgow Rent Strike was detached from 'the Labour campaign for municipal housing', how does this then explain the fact that, in 1918, when rent strike veterans Mrs Fergusson and Mrs Laird were included in the Local Government Board's (LGB) Women's Housing Committee, their report said:

> We think it right and necessary to express as an Addendum to our Report our opinion that before any real housing reform can be assured, it is imperative that the State should accept the principle that a proper standard of housing for the people is a national charge and a national concern.
>
> (LGB for Scotland, *Women's Housing Report*, 1918)

These women are *explicitly* advancing the labour campaign for municipal housing.

With regard to Castells' argument, the implication is that only when the proletariat is engaged in its final apocalyptic struggle to overthrow the bourgeoisie can we talk of 'class struggle'. The corollary is that the working class is wasting its time in any struggle which is not the final revolutionary overthrow of the capitalist state. Such a perspective overlooks the 'struggle for hegemony' which is continuously going on at every interstice of the social formation (Gramsci 1971). It also overlooks those aspects of the self-activation of the working class expressed in Clydeside revolutionary John Maclean's famous exhortation: 'Agitate! Educate! Organize!' Agitation, education and organization are vital aspects of the class struggle as it is precisely in this kind of self-activity that the working class can learn its political lessons, and raise its consciousness. It is for these reasons that I would argue that the 1915 Rent Strike, and the subsequent Rent and Mortgage Interest (War Restrictions) Act 1915, constituted a notable victory for the working class. Quite apart from the invaluable lessons in political organization learned in the course of these struggles, this claim is based on three separate factors: (i) the Rent Act protected working-class tenants from wartime exploitation of their house rents; (ii) it crystallized the necessity for state intervention in the working-class housing market in the post-war years; and (iii) it dealt a severe body blow to the urban bourgeoisie of Glasgow, that complex of lawyers, property-owners and factors[1] who effectively controlled the local state, and thus their working-class tenants.

Thus, Castells is talking nonsense when he argues that there was a lack of 'direct confrontation with the dominant faction [*sic*] of the capital' in the Glasgow working class of 1915. He is perpetrating an illegitimate separation of politics and economics. Assuming that he means dominant *fraction* of capital, it can readily be seen from the evidence that the fraction which the Glasgow tenants did *directly* confront in 1915 was that which was dominant in *their* lives, namely local rentier capital in the form of the landlords and factors of the city. Again, it is worth stressing the point that the working-class movement has to fight its class struggles where it stands, and not where academics twenty-five years on would have them fight with the benefit of hindsight. The working-class women of Glasgow and the ILP activists defined the central enemy in the Rent Strike as the landlords and factors, precisely located the chain of capital flow from bond-holders as the origin of the 'rent problem', and recommended radical, albeit reformist, state strategies to attack this problem. It does not matter that the 'housing crisis [was] a secondary contradiction under the conditions of early capitalism', as Castells argues (1983). It was one of *the* major contradictions in wartime Glasgow (and elsewhere in Britain), and by taking autonomous action, the local working class levered open more contradictions, not only on the material level of state policy towards rent control and council housing, but also on the ideological level in terms of notions of what was acceptable to the working class's own living standards. This in turn led to a protracted and bitter defence of the 1915 gains in Clydebank, as we shall see, while all of these struggles, offensive or defensive, constituted a challenge to the hegemony of the local urban bourgeoisie.

Saunders' position is equally tenuous. There are many instances of localized struggles in Britain which have had outcomes at the level of the state. One has only to think of 'Poplarism', the unemployed struggles of the inter-war years, the 1981 Black uprising, and the anti-poll tax campaign in Scotland – episodes of struggle which are considered elsewhere in this volume. I have argued that the 1915 Glasgow Rent Strike was one such struggle, and will argue here that the 1920s Clydebank Rent Strike was another. There is a very important sense in which the demands of these rent strikers became incorporated in subsequent housing legislation, and indeed within the welfare state itself. These were struggles which prefigured issues that were later seen as 'normal' components of mass democracy; in other words, they constituted quintessential 'struggles for hegemony'.

It can be seen, then, that the assumptions behind Castells' and Saunders' arguments lead to a pernicious situation characterized thus by John Foster in a critique of Castells:

> They sunder just those relationships which are the most crucial ones. The flux of language and cultural identity is abstracted from its immediate social determinants. Above all, the individual – albeit the social individual – is no longer seen as the focus and expression of the contradictions of a mode of production as a social system.
>
> (Foster 1979: 110)

Precisely. Castells, Melling and Saunders all posit the state as some kind of phenomenon 'up in the sky', as something which is abstract and detached from people's lives. But in the late twentieth century, the state has never been more important in terms of interfering in people's immediate personal, social and political lives. It is continuously developing new forms of surveillance, control and domination which are *very* apparent at the local level, whether through the Education or Health Authorities, the Council Tax Office, the Housing and Social Work Departments, probation officers and the police, the Inland Revenue or Benefits Agency, to name but a few.

I shall now turn to the Clydebank Rent Strike of the 1920s to see if further sense can be made of such local struggles. Why? A pioneering article on rent strikes makes the following important point:

> One reason for examining forms of direct political action such as squatting or withholding rent is that, unlike voting behaviour, they are likely to be highly significant for those involved; they

demand of participants not only involvement in illegal behaviour but also a normative commitment quite different from that necessary to sustain the ritualistic placing of a cross on a ballot paper every four or five years.

(Moorhouse *et al.* 1972: 138)

As we shall see, the Clydebank Rent Strike was highly significant for the people involved, who evinced a degree of 'normative commitment' to it which was quite remarkable.

'The Clyde Rent War!'[2]

The origins of the Clydebank Rent Strike lie firmly in the Glasgow Rent Strike of 1915, which should more properly be called the 'Clydeside Rent Strike', as it affected towns throughout Clydeside, from Airdrie to Greenock. In the famous confrontation with Glasgow Sheriff Lee,[3] on 17 November 1915, delegates from the Clydebank shipyards had been the most militant advocates of the rent strikers' case (Damer 1980: 99). Indeed, as early as April 1915, the Clydebank Trades Council had proposed a demonstration against the rent increases and the establishment of a Fair Rents Tribunal (*Minutes*, 2 February 1915 and 5 February 1915). Thus, when the Rent and Mortgage Interest (Restrictions) Act 1920 proposed a 10 per cent increase over the 'standard' rent (the rent level of 1914) of controlled houses, with a further 25 per cent increase if essential repairs were carried out, the tenants of Clydebank – and Glasgow – were furious, as *no* repairs or maintenance, essential or otherwise, had been carried out since the start of the war. The Clydebank Town Council unanimously passed a resolution which viewed 'with grave concern the indignation and discontent of the tenants in this vicinity caused by the Government's proposed Increase of Rent Bill' (*Clydebank Press*, 25 June 1920).

The National Conference of the Scottish Labour Housing Association held a meeting in Glasgow on 5 August 1920 which was attended by 1,000 delegates representing 400 organizations from all over Scotland; John Wheatley, the ILP's housing expert, was chair. A 24-hour general strike was proposed on 23 August 1920 in protest against the Rent Act and was approved unanimously by the delegates (*Clydebank Press*, 6 August 1920). The strike took place with mass support and demonstrations in both Clydebank and Glasgow. In both places, resolutions against paying the increased rent were passed, and the Notices of Increase of Rent were made into piles and burned

(*Clydebank Press*, 27 August 1920). However, in spite of these resolutions, when rent day came there was no organized resistance in Glasgow, with the *Glasgow Herald* reporting that the factors and their clerks were collecting the increased rent without difficulty. However, in Clydebank, when the factors asked for the full rent – the standard rent and the permitted 10 per cent increase – they were offered only the standard rent. Some factors took the money as an instalment against the full rent, writing-up the balance as arrears, while others refused to accept anything except the full amount (*Clydebank Press*, 3 September 1920).

Thus, from the very beginning of the operations of the Rent Restrictions Act 1920, Clydebank tenants were refusing to pay anything more than the 'standard rent', rent at the level obtaining in 1914. It should also be noted that all over Clydeside, the Scottish Labour Housing Association, through its local branches, was orchestrating the resistance to rent increases, and the resolutions passed at different meetings in different areas tended to be identical. Messrs Wheatley, Kirkwood and MacBride, and Mrs Laird and Mrs Dollan, prominent ILP housing activists, were the central figures in the Association at this time. Two questions remain: (i) what were the grounds of resistance to the increases? and (ii) why was there mass resistance in Clydebank and not in Glasgow?

The answer to the first question was one of socialist political principle, and the hand of John Wheatley, the ILP's housing expert, can clearly be seen at work. The argument was a compounded one whereby (a) working people could not afford the increases in rent; (b) even if they could afford the increase they should not have to pay as the houses they lived in were generally unfit for human habitation; (c) people should not be allowed to make profit out of such housing; and (d) the obligation was on the state to build decent houses for the working class, as required by the Housing and Town Planning Act 1919, through Direct Labour schemes. Remembering that the Scottish Labour Housing Association was a creation of the ILP, it is this complex of class-based arguments which gives the lie to Melling's claim that the rent strikes were in some sense 'autonomous' from the working-class movement, or Castells' position that they constituted an autonomous 'urban social movement', or Saunders' argument that they were merely 'social consumption' struggles.

The answer to the second question is less obvious, and must remain somewhat speculative without further research. But the most plausible hypothesis as to why the 1920s Rent Strike took off in Clydebank lies in its distinctive labour and housing markets, and the strong links between the two. Thus, paralleling the 1915 situation in Glasgow where the Rent Strike was most solid in the shipbuilding areas of Partick and Govan (Damer 1980; Melling 1983), political organization in Clydebank in the 1920s was strongest in the areas containing co-workers from the same unit of production – Radnor Park, for example, where the workers in the giant Singer's plant were concentrated. And, obviously, the radical socialist climate of the town was the background to this and subsequent political action. There was an identifiable cadre of ILP and Scottish Labour Party (SLP) – and later, Communist Party – families in Clydebank, almost constituting a separate 'estate'. One could live one's whole life in this milieu, learning one's class politics before reaching school age. Finally, Clydebank was geographically much smaller and more compact than Glasgow.

1920 ended with two highly significant Sheriff Court cases involving the rent issue: first in Glasgow, and then in Clydebank. A legal challenge was made with regard to the legality of the factors' Notices of Increase of Rent. The case hinged on highly technical matters known as 'Tacit Relocation' in Scottish law, which I have discussed at length elsewhere (Damer 1982; 1985), but matters which the Clydeside activists soon mastered. They argued that factors had to issue what was known as a 'Notice of Removal' before they could issue a Notice of Increase of Rent. On 15 September 1920, Councillor Emmanuel Shinwell appeared before the Glasgow Sheriff Court after refusing to pay a rent increase on these grounds. The Glasgow Sheriff rejected Shinwell's defence, and he was evicted from his home. This judgment constituted the legal precedent in cases of this nature in Glasgow.

In the second case, on 26 November 1920 in Dunbartonshire Sheriff Court – which covered Clydebank – Sheriff-Substitute Menzies held that rent increases permitted by the 1920 Act 'are invalid where no terminating Notice has been issued' and 'that any excess rent paid beyond the Standard Rent is recoverable right back to 1915' (*Glasgow Herald*, 26 November 1920). This sensational judgment was completely at variance with the Glasgow Sheriff Court ruling, and was immediately seized on by the Clydebank branch of the Scottish Labour Housing Association who mounted a campaign based on the ruling. The Clyde Rent War had begun in earnest.

However, for the rest of 1920 and throughout 1921 the war was a phoney one; the situation on Clydeside, particularly in Clydebank, was stalemate. *De jure*, the factors were entitled to a 10 per cent increase, *de facto*, they were not getting it. From the evidence of contemporary newspapers like the *Glasgow Herald* and the *Clydebank Press*, it would appear that local sheriffs were loath to grant eviction decrees if there was any hope of even token instalments towards the arrears being paid. The issue, particularly in Clydebank, was hardly one of the factors getting the increased rent, rather, it was a case of them getting even the standard rent. However, the human cost of this endless litigation against poor people is caught in this poetic passage from the usually anti-working class newspaper, the *Glasgow Herald*:

> The court-room was crowded, and the passages were thronged with people who were waiting for their cases to be called. Their appearance gave a somewhat vivid impression of the distress prevailing in the city. Most of then were poorly clad, and not a few showed traces of the pinch of poverty. There were women wearing shawls and carrying children in their arms, and bent old men who seemed to find the climb up the stairs to the court-room a tax on their strength. Here and there could be seen disabled men with crutches, and a large proportion of the crowd were unemployed, as the subsequent proceedings in the court showed. ... About 300 decrees for ejection were granted.
>
> (*Glasgow Herald*, 2 July 1921)

1922 started with the Dumbarton ILP solicitor, D. D. Cormack, winning a series of eviction cases for Clydebank tenants on the 'Invalid Notice' plea. A week later, the Dumbarton Sheriff-Substitute held that *all* the Notices of Increase issued by the Glasgow Property Owners and Factors Association (GPOFA) (whose members factored the Clydebank tenements) were invalid on this legal point, but that a test case was needed to decide the matter. At the same time, the Annual Conference of the Scottish Labour Housing Association passed a resolution that the working class would make sure the house of any evictee would not be reoccupied by a new tenant. The Clydeside socialists may not have been expert analysts of international monopoly capital, but they certainly knew how to recognize their immediate enemy.

The test case was hastily heard on 25 March 1922, and became famous as *Kerr* v. *Bryde*. A factor, Kerr, took his tenant Dugald Bryde before Sheriff-Substitute Menzies in Dumbarton for eviction on the grounds of arrears of rent. The arrears were in respect of unpaid increases of rent. The lawyer for the defence, D. D. Cormack, argued that the Notice of Increase was invalid because a Notice to Quit had not been served first. Sheriff Menzies found in favour of Bryde and dismissed the case.

The GPOFA promptly appealed to the Sheriff Principal who upheld his subordinate's decision (*Clydebank Press*, 28 April 1922). The GPOFA appealed again, this time to the Court of Session in Edinburgh. On 30 June, to the horror of the factors, the Court of Session upheld the Dumbarton sheriffs' decisions (*Glasgow Herald*, 26 June 1922). An immediate consequence was that the Glasgow sheriffs announced they would not consider decrees for eviction unless tenants were at least nine months in arrears with their rent (*GPOFA Annual Report* 1923: 3). The GPOFA then took its case to the House of Lords. The hearing started on 18 July, and the almost indecent haste with which the hearing was arranged did not go unremarked in Clydebank (*Clydebank Press*, 15 September 1922). However, the Law Lords postponed issuing judgment until the autumn diet as the run-up to a general election was in full swing. They finally issued their judgment on 2 November 1922, upholding the previous court's decision in favour of the tenant. The party in Clydebank, like that in Glasgow on the announcement of the Rent and Mortgage Interest (War Restrictions) Act 1915, went on all night. The decision was a calamity for the GPOFA, but proved to be of vital importance for the local working-class community.

Both sides to the dispute reacted quickly, but it was Labour who fired the first shot. On 6 November 1922, in the same issue in which the *Glasgow Herald* carried an interview with the City Assessor on the possible consequences of the House of Lords' decision – in theory, £3 million in paid-up increases in rent was owed to tenants – the Scottish Labour Housing Association issued a manifesto. As a result of the *Kerr* v. *Bryde* decision, tenants could reclaim a sum equal to twelve months' rent and rates, and the Association would advise them on how to go about collecting the money. On 9 November, ILP candidate David Kirkwood pledged his support for standard-rent-only at a public ILP general election meeting held at Clydebank Town Hall. He was quoted as saying: 'those who voted for Mr. Taylor [the sitting MP] had to remember that every vote cast for him was a vote cast for the Factor and a continuance of the awful conditions that prevailed in Clydebank at the moment' (*Clydebank Press*, 10 November 1922).

It does not take a very profound reading of the contemporary regional and national press to realize that all the Scottish ILP candidates in the election made the rent issue a central plank in their platforms, for example Stewart in St Rollox, Maxton in Bridgeton, McDougall in Tradeston, Kirkwood in Dumbarton Burghs (which included Clydebank) and Wheatley in Shettleston, *inter alia*. Nothing could stop the avalanche. The ILP swept through Clydeside and ten

'Red Clydeside' MPs were elected for Glasgow City alone, with David Kirkwood running away with Dumbarton Burghs with a 7,290 majority. It is salutary to remember what class hatred can be like. Following the election, the *Glasgow Herald* had this to say:

> We cannot view without profound dissatisfaction the significant gains made by Labour in industrial Scotland and most conspicuously in the Glasgow constituencies. ... The lesson writ large over the electoral returns is that Labour, notwithstanding the incongruous elements it may include and the natural tendencies it would display to split under the strains and stresses of responsible administration, is for fighting purposes a united and formidably organised body skilfully addressing itself to class prejudice and to individual cupidity – emotions, passions and desires far more potent than those which the commonplaces of the ordinary politician can arouse. ... It is certainly easier in this country to create a mass of socialists by depressing the standards of morality than it is to keep the majority to sound ideas of citizenship.
>
> (*Glasgow Herald*, 17 November 1922)

For once, however, the *Herald* was right: the ILP, and its constituent bodies like the Scottish Labour Housing Association, *was* a 'formidably organised body' addressing itself not to 'class prejudice', but to class *analysis*. It is considerations like this which make the arguments of Castells, Melling and Saunders so tendentious.

The new year started with a clarion call by the 1923 Annual Conference of the Scottish Labour Housing Association (with all the Scottish Labour MPs present and 3,000 delegates) for defence of the gains represented by the *Kerr* v. *Bryde* decision, for an overall return to 1914 rents, and for a campaign against eviction of tenants for arrears of rent arising from unemployment or low wages. Significantly, it also added a call (from the Glasgow Trades Council) for the immediate construction of the half a million council houses pledged under the Housing Act 1919 programme, and for the release of Treasury funds to subsidize the rents of these houses at average local levels (*Glasgow Herald*, 3 January 1923).

In Clydebank, four ILP councillors had been elected plus Andrew Leiper as an Independent. Leiper was the organizer of the Clydebank Labour Housing Association branch and a central, if ambiguous, player in the Rent Strike (see Damer 1982). While it is impossible to give an accurate figure, from an analysis of contemporary newspapers it would seem that thousands of Clydebank tenants were on rent strike by the beginning of 1923. Some people refused to pay the increased rent but tendered the standard rent. Some tenants put aside the difference between the standard and the increased rent in case of a reversal of the *Kerr* v. *Bryde* decision, but other tenants spent the money. Times were hard. Some tenants refused to pay any rent until the legal situation had been clarified; meanwhile, some clearly took advantage of the situation and abandoned the idea of paying rent altogether. The factors exacerbated the situation by not having an agreed policy among themselves: some took the standard rent, some would take only the increased rent, while others would take payment by instalment.

There was a great deal of state anxiety. The Interim Report of the Committee on Housing Policy (January 1923) highlighted a central contradiction in government thinking:

> Assuming, as they must assume, that a proposal for the continuance temporarily of the Rent Restriction Act will have to be made in Parliament, the Committee does not see how the Government, while thus admitting shortage of housing accommodation, can at the same time repudiate the responsibility of doing anything to mitigate that shortage during the period of the extension of the Act.
>
> (CP 8(23) in CAB 27/208)

On 5 February 1923, the Onslow Committee on the Rent Restriction Act 1920 reported its findings (Cmd., 1803, 1923). In brief, it recommended the removal of restriction as soon as possible, but it also admitted that, for the immediate future, this was not a politically viable option. It further recommended that the rent increases allowed under the 1920 Act be continued. The bill which the Government subsequently introduced into Parliament produced an uproar from the Labour side as it was proposed that the increases in rent be made payable retrospectively from 1 December 1922. Thus the direct action of Clydebank tenants had produced a most unusual parliamentary precedent: retrospective legislation.

The Annual Report of the GPOFA summarized the situation at the beginning of the year:

> The legislation proposed was, that what a tenant had retained or deducted prior to 1st December 1922 he was to retain in respect of his claim for repayment of invalid increases since August 1920. Where the tenant had paid the increased rent in full up to 1st

December he was to lose all right to retain. The Bill further provided that all arrears of invalidated increases since 1st December 1922 and up to 15th February 1923, along with all arrears of rent retained by the tenant between these dates, were to be payable by instalments at the rate of 20 per cent of the standard rent, along with periodical rent payments. Subject to these exceptions, the statutory Notices were declared to have been valid *ab initio*, and any statutory Notices for the future were to be deemed to have effect as if they were also Notice to terminate the existing tenancy.

(*GPOFA Annual Report* 1924: 2)

The period for paying by instalments was in fact increased under Labour pressure in committee to the date of the passing of the Act, and the percentage of the standard rent as the criterion for the repayment of these instalments was cut from 20 to 15 per cent.

The Act, which appeared in June, satisfied no one. It did not give the factors all the increases they wanted, but it did allow increases which the tenants did not want. This compromise served to strengthen the Rent Strike. By allowing those who had not paid to keep part of their rent money, and by allowing the landlords to keep all of the increased rent from those who had paid, the government strengthened the resolve of first, those who had paid to withhold their rent in the future, and second, those who had not paid to continue to withhold their rent. As early as January 1924, David Kirkwood was calling on his constituents to 'pay no rent', and to raise 'home guards' against eviction (Damer 1985: 24). It was only a matter of time before the factors would resort to their traditional weapon: eviction.

At this juncture, it should be made clear that the oral history of the Clydebank Rent Strike demonstrates that local working-class tenants knew precisely the legal situation, and they had already established a town-wide defence system comprising of (a) look-outs from the National Unemployed Workers Movement (NUWM) who patrolled the Clydebank borders by bicycle on the scout for the Sheriff Officers and their men; and (b) groups of housewives organized on a close[4] and street basis, ready to drop everything to resist the eviction of a neighbour. The latter signalled the presence of the detested Sheriff Officers by ringing brass handbells bought specially for the purpose. This oral evidence has been presented elsewhere, but a couple of short extracts will demonstrate the sophistication of both the legal knowledge and the organizational skills of working-class Clydebank tenants (Damer 1985: 25–6). (Mr Lambie was a 23-year-old unemployed semi-skilled worker and ex-serviceman in 1922):

LAMBIE: The Rent Strike started as a result of the evictions – the eviction decrees that the landlords were starting to take to Court. The 1920 Act laid it down that where a valid Notice to Quit was sent, the landlord had the right to impose a new contract, he was entitled to increase his rent. But he had to terminate his old contract first. So they put up their defence: 'No Valid Notice to Quit – Kerr versus Bryde'. And auld Dugald Bryde was an old, old man doon one o' the side streets doon by Bon Accord Street. But that case went right on and on until it went to the House of Lords, and we won!

DAMER: What was the case about?

L: In the 1920s increase, they couldn't increase the rent unless they terminated the contractual tenancy that existed by 'Tacit Relocation' ... an agreement existed and by Tacit Relocation it kept on and on until terminated. And the termination medium was a Notice to Quit.

D: Yes. Which had to be legally valid?

L: Yes. A Valid Notice. So the first defence was 'No Valid Notice'. And the Kerr versus Bryde case went on from there.

Yet another eyewitness had this to say on the resistance to evictions:

> as soon as it became known, the people concerned, or the neighbours, weren't long in raising the alarm when an eviction was to take place. They knew in advance in most cases when it was taking place. And if there were sufficient time they got the band out – the band attached to the NUWM. We rounded up as many of the band as we could at short notice, and marched to the scene of the eviction. ... And when the Sheriff's Officers came along to carry out the evictions the house was crammed. And they were unable to get in.
>
> (McCafferty, in Damer 1985)

The Clydebank Rent Strike was by now a national *cause célèbre*, meriting leaders in *The Times*, regular and acerbic parliamentary exchanges, and, of course, serving as a source of fury in the GPOFA, which estimated that 12,000 Clydebank tenants were on rent strike (*The Times*, 5 September 1924). It was all rather impressive given that, in the view of Castells, Melling and Saunders, thousands of working-class people were not only *not* engaged in hand-to-hand combat with the dominant fraction of capital, but also, they were not even engaged in *class* struggle.

The situation deteriorated throughout 1924. The Secretary for Scotland, Willie Adamson, a right-winger, made several visits to Clydebank to negotiate with the factors and the Housing Association. It is at this point that we can begin to see a shift in the politics of the Rent Strike. At the end of March 1924, John Wheatley had tried to produce a bill to prevent evictions. This was talked out in the notorious fiasco (Marquand 1977: 321ff.). Given the various pressures on the Labour Party, and the later introduction of Wheatley's own Housing Bill, it is hardly surprising that this particular issue did not receive any more parliamentary time. The best that could be done under the circumstances was to fight to continue rent control.

Further, in Parliament Tory MPs openly accused the 'Red Clyde-side' MPs in general, and David Kirkwood in particular, of fomenting lawlessness in Clydebank. They had already been labelled 'the wild men from the Clyde' by *The Times*, which had also been responsible in 1919 for coining the term 'the Red Clyde'. Matters were not helped by the intransigence of Andrew Leiper and his colleagues in the Clydebank Housing Association. Although a constituent branch of the Scottish Labour Housing Association, Leiper (as organizer) insisted that it was a 'non-party' organization. This earned him a great deal of criticism from local socialists, and alienated him from the ILP, not to mention the Communist Party militants in the NUWM. Furthermore, he had organized a 'rent control' fund into which he encouraged striking tenants to pay standard rent which was then banked. Local activists again attacked this as a counter-productive tactic, arguing that rent increases of one kind or another were inevitable, and that these funds could be seized at law by the factors to pay off arrears. The people who hated Leiper most, however, were the factors. It was his intransigent call for a global return to standard rents, and no negotiation, which infuriated them. Even worse, and most curiously in terms of his insistence that the Housing Association was 'non-party', was his demand that the municipality, or the state, 'expropriate' all the Clydebank tenements as the factors were unable or unwilling to manage them on behalf of the people. As this was effectively a revolutionary demand, it can be seen that his notion of 'non-party' did not mean 'non-political'. In the event, Adamson could wring no changes out of the Association, the factors were preparing for mass evictions, and the ILP was thoroughly embarrassed.

Clydebank Town Council was also embarrassed. The Burgh was over £24,000 in rates arrears for 1924 which the factors had refused, or said they were unable to pay because the tenants were paying little or no rent. A committee, organized by the Town Council and including representatives from both sides – tenants and factors – was not working. Towards the end of 1924 *The Times* made the comment that: 'Communist influence on Clydebank, working on a population which is largely of Irish origin, have [*sic*] contrived to keep the Rent Strike alive' (17 November 1924). The paper also carried two photographs of evictions in Clydebank, demonstrating the importance of this issue to the ruling class.

The remaining three years of the Rent Strike (1925–7) saw the state chip away at the Clydebank tenants' legal position, while locally the factors stepped-up evictions only to be met by more and more determined resistance. In January 1925, the government appointed a Commission under Lord Constable:

> To enquire and report on the economic and other difficulties in carrying out the provisions of the Rent Restriction Acts which have arisen in some districts of Scotland, with a view to more efficient working during the continuation of said Acts, and to simplification of procedure under them.
>
> (Committee on the Rent Restriction Act, 1925: 1)

Much play had been made in Parliament by David Kirkwood of the fact that Clydebank tenants were not paying the increased rent because they could not afford it. The Commission took Kirkwood at his word. Mr Cunnison, an economist at the University of Glasgow, undertook a study of Clydebank and Port Glasgow to determine the living conditions there. He had already conducted a similar study in Anderston in Glasgow. Family incomes in all three areas were low, but rents in Clydebank were much higher than in Anderston, and somewhat higher than in Port Glasgow. The trouble in interpreting the survey data lay in the fact that the three areas were not strictly comparable. In the event, one finding emerged clearly: 'there is nothing in the present economic conditions of Clydebank, compared with other places, to justify or explain the extraordinary differences which exist between them in the payment of rent and rates' (Cmd., 2423, 1925: 22). The problem lay, the Report continued, in the 'persistent litigation' in which the Clydebank tenants indulged in the Sheriff Court. Comparing Clydebank to the rest of the region, it continued:

> The tension between factors and tenants is greater; the tenants are better organised; and propagandism has not been without effect. But we do not think that organisation and propagandism would

have availed unless they had been recommended by legal success
in defeating the operation of the Acts.

(Ibid.: 22)

The Report found that there was a spirit of conciliation in the air;
many tenants were confused as to how much and what rent they owed.
The Report refers to several councillors and officials of the local ILP
agreeing to the need to stop the endless 'dog-fighting', while the point
was made that in these times of unemployment owners must be
prepared to make some sacrifices, and especially, those who were
unemployed should not have 'severe measures' taken against them.

The recommendations of the Report were essentially that an
amending statute be passed to refer to Scotland alone, and this should
simplify the procedure of the Notice of Increase of Rent (Cmd., 2423
1925: 22, para. 39). There should be a time limit to the period allowed
for objections by the tenant, but the factor should be required to
supply all details of the increase on application by the tenant, and this
should be checked by a Town Council official. The court should be
directed to take into account exceptional hardship of tenants, and
accordingly the courts should be given the power to suspend or
discharge eviction decrees. Rent books should be standardized and a
committee should be formed in Clydebank to mediate between
landlords and tenants.

Paddy Dollan, an ILP councillor and parliamentary candidate,
issued a lengthy minority Report which disagreed in emphasis with the
majority Report, but did agreed that a new Act should be passed to
put an end to the litigation. He wanted rent control continued for
another ten years and the rents of controlled houses immediately
reduced by 25 per cent. He also wanted strong local authority control
over the condition of private property. It is worth noting that several
Clydebank tenants, in giving evidence to the Commission, reported
that they simply could not afford the rents. They estimated that it took
£3 9s 0d a week to feed a family of four, while the Old Kilpatrick
Parish Council (which covered Clydebank) allowance for a family of
four was £1 14s 6d a week – the highest in Scotland (*Clydebank Press*,
6 March 1925).

The GPOFA saw the Constable Commission's Report as a vindica-
tion of their case, and began slowly to step up the rate of evictions.
Andrew Leiper agreed with Paddy Dollan's recommendation for a 25
per cent reduction in the rents of controlled houses, but questioned
how this was to be achieved. The Clydebank Town Council had a
stormy meeting to discuss the Report which led to Leiper and the

Housing Association representatives walking out. The meeting was deeply divided, with various contradictory resolutions, recriminations and arguments about tactics being aired (*Clydebank Press*, 15 February 1925). It seems clear that from this point the Rent Strike began to fade. Towards the end of the year, the factors began to step up the rate of evictions. By November, Leiper was using Sheriff Menzies' 'rule of court' in eviction cases, whereby there was a continuation to permit the tenant to make some deal with the factor (*Clydebank Press*, 13 November 1925). In the same month, in the municipal elections, the ILP was ousted in Clydebank and Andrew Leiper lost his seat as an Independent.

The *coup de grâce* for the tenants' morale came at the beginning of December when the *Clydebank Press* printed an abject and crawling letter from MacAlpine's tenants in the 'Holy City' (the Radnor Park Housing Estate, Clydebank) pledging to do their utmost to pay arrears in rent *and* the increased rent. MacAlpine's lawyer accepted the tenants' offer but imposed crippling conditions (*Clydebank Press*, 14 December 1925). Many people saw this as a sell-out by the tenants, and this produced bitter recriminations, including a letter from Leiper attacking the tenants, and subsequent counter-letters attacking him. The factors rubbed in their victory by evicting six families on 31 December – Hogmanay – and met no resistance. The only respite was that, as yet, no new Rent Act had been passed following on the Constable Report, although a bill had received one reading.

More Byzantine legal wrangling continued during 1926. None the less, by the end of 1926 and the beginning of 1927 Leiper was still winning cases for both individual tenants and slates of tenants before Sheriff-Substitute Menzies. However, the factors of Singers' property resorted to an underhand tactic: they went for arrestment of wages to collect their arrears of rent. Then, on 21 July, Andrew Leiper was accidentally knocked down by a car in Clydebank. He died in the Glasgow Western Infirmary on 9 August (*Clydebank Press*, 22 July 1927). The GPOFA seized the opportunity to announce what it believed to be the end of the Clydebank Housing Association, and promptly served 48-hours Notice to Quit on a large number of tenants in the Radnor Park area, the heart of the Rent Strike, and where the Singers' workers lived (*Clydebank Press*, 19 August 1927).

At about the same time, a critical decision was made in yet another appeal to the Court of Session. In the Marshall case, as it was called, the tenant had not been paying the increase on standard rent on the grounds that the wording on the Notice of Increase forms was legally invalid (*Clydebank Press*, 15 July 1927). The court, however, ruled that the Notices were as valid as it was possible to make them, and called upon sheriffs to interpret the law 'benignly and not malignantly'. This Jesuitical judgment constituted a nod as good as a wink to a liberal sheriff.

This can be considered the end of the Rent Strike. It should not be forgotten that the wider context of this particular struggle was the national defeat of the 1926 General Strike and general demoralization within the working-class movement. However, the Housing Association was not yet finished, and it continued to fight cases, including yet another appeal to the Court of Session, until at least the end of 1927. The NUWM continued to fight rent cases for its own members right up until the 1930s, although the bulk of these actions were involved with negotiating settlements for tenants on arrears of rent (Damer 1982: 22).

Needless to say, the GPOFA wreaked its vengeance on the militant rent strikers. Many of the leaders of the Rent Strike were evicted, and one family wound up living in a tent in the Clydebank municipal park throughout the winter of 1927/28, while others lived in converted railway wagons (Damer 1982: 25). Mr Lambie, Andrew Leiper's lieutenant, was effectively blacklisted in Clydebank, and had to leave town with his family to seek a new life in England. Others, similarly shamed by the stigma of eviction, quietly vanished from Clydebank. Local militancy about the rents issue subsided. The *political issue* of controlled rents, however, refused to go away.

The Clydebank Rent Strike: a working-class struggle?

What, in a theoretical sense, are we to make of the Clydebank Rent Strike? Was it a success or a failure? Was it an episode of the class struggle, or some kind of residual 'urban struggle', or struggle over 'social consumption'? Presumably, Castells, Melling and Saunders would all argue that, like the 1915 Glasgow Rent Strike, the Clydebank Rent Strike was *not* a class struggle because the strikers did not man the barricades or propose a revolutionary transition. Presumably, they would also argue that in the long term the strikers lost because the courts finally ruled against the tenants, many of the leaders were evicted, and a central demand – that of the maintenance of the 1914 level of rent – was not achieved. This position, I would argue, is naïve.

In capitalist society, class struggle is happening continuously in every interstice of the social formation. Sometimes this struggle is open and spectacular, more often, though, it is less dramatic and barely visible and is waged on an ideological plane. Before the First World

War, as I have shown definitively elsewhere (Damer 1980), working-class tenants in Scotland were at the mercy of laws which exclusively protected the interests of the property-owning class, and left them at the mercy of the factors, the agents of that class. And the factors were merciless. The 1915 Glasgow Rent Strike successfully challenged the local hegemony of the GPOFA.

The essence of capitalist society is class struggle and class oppression. The working-class's tactical defence of its rights, and its tactical offensive against the bourgeoisie will be limited to what is historically available in both material and ideological terms. When one considers that the years of the Clydebank Rent Strike (1920–7) were the years of the Depression, and included the calamity of the 1926 General Strike, then the two-pronged strategy of the Clydebank tenants – fighting the factors at law, on the one hand, and resisting evictions by civil disobedience, on the other – was strikingly imaginative. This strategy led to gains for local tenants in three key areas: (i) immediate material gains; (ii) immediate and long-term political gains in the form of parliamentary representation for themselves and the Scottish working class; and (iii) long-term effects on the issue of the politics of the social reproduction of the working class in housing. Let us consider each of these gains in turn.

The Rent Strike achieved a considerable degree of material success in so far as very large numbers of Clydebank tenants paid only standard rent, or less, from 1920 right up to, and in some cases beyond, 1927. (The GPOFA's own estimate of rent strikers was 12,000, as we have seen, although that figure may have been inflated for political reasons.) Further, both during and after the Rent Strike, settlements – deals – were explicitly encouraged by the Dumbarton Sheriff Court. Clearly, some tenants would have been bullied into paying some or all of their arrears, but whether this number was large is doubtful. The factors had to face the reality of mass unemployment, and clearly, some rent money was better than none. Thus the tenants of Clydebank conducted an effective defence of their standard of living for a protracted period at a time of mass unemployment. While this may not impress Castells, Melling or Saunders, it certainly impressed the governments of the time, the courts, the property-owning class in general, and the GPOFA in particular.

Of course, it has to be admitted that the Clydebank tenants failed to export their Rent Strike, and Melling is correct when he notes that one reason for this is that it was not supported by the trade union movement, as was the case with the 1915 Glasgow Strike (Melling 1983). However, this argument is perhaps not as compelling as it might at first appear. In the first instance, the circumstances of the 1915 strike were unique: it occurred in the middle of a war. During the 1920s in Clydebank, there was no war, there was widespread local industrial unemployment, the working class was reeling after the defeat of the 1926 General Strike, and the trade union movement was busy looking after its own members. Further, this movement has only occasionally been centrally concerned with non-industrial struggles. And if the Clydebank tenants failed to export their strike, it was not for want of trying. Speakers were dispatched to every corner of Scotland. It is plain from sampling local newspapers that there were rent strikes, court cases and considerable agitation elsewhere, particularly in west central Scotland, and this requires further research. It is my impression that elsewhere in Scotland, sheriffs sat it out, waiting for a definitive ruling on the ambiguous Rent Acts. They were quite happy to let Sheriff-Substitute Menzies bear the brunt of the criticism for his liberal interpretation of the law.

The strategic legal issue was that the Rent Restriction Acts of 1915, and those of subsequent years, were intended at law to protect working-class tenants from landlords. This was what constituted a most important gain for the Scottish working class. This point was explicitly acknowledged by Lord Skerrington in his judgment on *Kerr* v. *Bryde*:

> the success of the action depends on the validity of the theory that an Act of Parliament primarily intended to protect the tenants ... from having their rents increased beyond what was permitted by statute ought to be construed as conferring upon the landlords the power of an unprecedented and anomalous description – the essence of which would deprive the tenant of a fundamental right.
> (SC 860, 1927: *Clydebank Investment Co. Ltd.* v. *Marshall*)

This 'fundamental and valuable right' was the continuation of a contractual tenancy by reason of Tacit Relocation. In this case, the judges were obliged to issue a relatively literal approach to the interpretation of the 1920 Rent Act. They could not hold that a fundamental principle of the common law of Scotland, i.e. Tacit Relocation, could be altered by implication in the 1920 Act. In other words, having won a legal right to have their rent controlled and tenancies protected by the legislation consequent upon the 1915 Rent Strike, the action of the Clydebank tenants won a reiteration and strengthening of that fundamental right in the judgment on the *Kerr* v. *Bryde* case. This was extremely important for Scottish tenants. For the state intended that that legislation should be temporary, as we have seen. Finance capital was exercising heavy pressure for its removal. The local struggles of the Clydebank tenants ensured that it became permanent. If they had remained silent, then that protection would have been removed.

The change in the legal struggle came after the factors began to follow the correct procedure for Notices – from about 1925 onwards – and formally terminated tenancies before issuing a Notice of Increase in Rent. This forced the Clydebank Housing Association away from arguments about legal *principle* towards arguments about legal *technicalities*. It was inevitable that the courts would issue a definitive judgment about these technicalities – in favour of the property-owners. The judges were able to fall back on the intention of the 1923 Rent Act – to increase rent. It is worth quoting Lord Anderson's judgment in the 1927 Marshall case at some length as he makes it perfectly plain what he is doing:

> These Acts of Parliament interfere with freedom of contract be-tween landlord and tenant; but for them the landlord would im-pose his own conditions of tenancy which the tenant would have to agree with or be without a house. They limit the freedom of contract which otherwise under the common law would be open to the landlord. ... Accordingly where a Sheriff-Substitute has to apply his mind to the construction of any of the statutory docu-ments such as, in this case, the Notice, he ought to construe that document benignly and not malignantly. And in the same way, when he is dealing with the actual language of the statute where it is ambiguous, the judge ought to construe the language reasona-bly and judicially and not judaically [*sic*] ... Sheriff-Substitutes dealing with these Acts of Parliament ought to do everything possible to discourage pleas in law which are based on mere tech-nicalities and which support no principle or consideration of justice.
>
> (*SC* 860 1927: *Clydebank Investment Co. Ltd.* v. *Marshall*)

Quite apart from the fact that Lord Anderson seems to have a different idea from the average tenant of what constitutes 'justice', what he is doing here is taking a more *interpretative* approach to the law – he was trying to make the Act work to give the factor his increase in rent. He was able to take a wider interpretation of the law as there was no issue of common law at stake – which was not the case in *Kerr* v. *Bryde*, where the judges were forced to take a more *literal* view of the law, in favour of the tenants. In 1927, the Law Lords were trying to simplify procedures for gaining the increases in rent, and negating the anomalous judgment in *Kerr* v. *Bryde*. However, the political climate had changed between 1920 and 1927 such that, while the Law Lords can be said to have won the battle, they effectively lost the war. The struggles of the Clydebank tenants had ensured that the whole issue of rents had moved on beyond the level of mere legal definition to the political arena – that of the state. And the state had learned its lesson; rent control remained on the statute books. It is this sort of real political outcome which makes the arguments of Saunders *et al.* so nugatory.

A final word about the women of Clydebank: let them not be hidden from history. It is plain that their internal social networks were central in the resistance to eviction, just as they were in 1915. These self-help networks, based on the close, were admirably adapted to rapid mobilization against the Sheriff Officers. Even in cases where evictions were successful, women either reinstated their neighbours in the houses from which they had just been evicted or took them into their own homes. Because of local women's responsibilities for budgeting within the gender division of labour, the rents issue was vital to the domestic economy at a time of large-scale unemployment. The longer they paid low – or no – rent, the better the women were able to manage the almost impossible job of feeding and clothing a family on the parish dole. Fortunately, the oral history of some of these women is told elsewhere (see Damer 1982).

These gains and losses are local empirical matters. What is more important is what were the class outcomes of this local class struggle? In the first instance, it formed the launching pad from which the Clydeside ILP MPs were shot into Parliament. These men remained for years the socialist conscience of the parliamentary Labour Party. They were tireless in defending the interests of their class, and John Wheatley's Housing Act of 1924 stands as a major stepping stone to the provision of state housing for the working class. The provision of many thousands of decent council houses may not impress Castells, Melling or Saunders, but it certainly impressed their working-class tenants.

In class terms, the other major gain of the Clydebank Rent Strike was to shift both the material and ideological terrain on which the battle over the cost of the social reproduction of the working class was fought. It was not just that rent control of small houses was continued. It was not just that a series of Housing Acts began to alleviate the scandalous housing conditions of large sections of the working class. It was that through their own struggles over the literal costs of their own lives, the local working class conceived of a new deal for itself in housing terms, and became conscious of a future in which the norm would not be an overcrowded and unhealthy slum, but a house with sufficient bedrooms, with a bathroom, with running water, and with a garden – at a fair rent, subsidized by the state. In other words, this struggle had an impact on social welfare and housing *policy*. The Clydebank Rent Strike was not the only working-class struggle in this process, but it was a vital one. It is the contention of this writer that but for this strike, rent control would have been removed by the mid-1920s.

Conclusion

It is obvious to anyone with an eye to hard data that so-called 'urban' or 'consumption' struggles are but facets of the overall class struggle. While they may not be directly related to struggles over the immediate process of production – or at least, not at first sight – this does not mean that they are not class struggles. The way to theorize these struggles is to locate them in the process of social reproduction, and the class struggle over reproduction and social welfare issues – rent, housing, health, education – is as bitter, if not more bitter, than struggles at the point of production. Historically, as well as in contemporary times, these struggles are deeply inimical to the interests of capital. The Clydebank Rent Strike was firmly located in the radical labourism of the Clydeside ILP. As Dave Byrne has observed: 'Labourism is not revolutionary consciousness, but the cultural context is deeply contradictory to capitalist social relations, especially and indeed fundamentally in the context of crisis' (1982: 73).

It is this cultural context and these social relations which Castells, Melling and Saunders seek to deny. The working-class movement on Clydeside was so well grounded in its cultural roots, and so well and fluidly organized, that it could encompass grass-roots rents struggles, theorize them in class terms offering a socialist critique of the capitalist housing market, fight it out in head-on confrontation with local rentier capital, and tie it all into a far-reaching campaign for municipal housing and fair rents in a manner which was comprehensible to local working people. This bespeaks an ability to theorize the workings of Clydeside rentier capital at a level of sophistication possibly too elegant for Castells, Melling and Saunders to comprehend. As John Wheatley observed:

if private enterprise could have given you clean or healthy cities and a healthy people, you would have nothing but healthy clean cities and healthy people because you have never had anything *but* private enterprise ... Private enterprise has given you your slums and rickety people. ... It has destroyed millions of the most useful and productive sections of our population.

(Glasgow Eastern Standard, 16 June 1923: 5)

Notes

1   A factor is an agent who collects rent and carries out repairs on behalf of property owners.
2   'The Clyde Rent War!' is the title of an ILP pamphlet by Paddy Dollan. It was a reprint of his Minority Report to the 1925 Constable Commission on the Rent Strike (see p. 87).
3   A Scottish sheriff is a judge roughly equivalent to an English county court judge, but with a much wider range of duties and powers.
4   A close is a common entrance stair to a tenement block.

6 The making of a poor people's movement

A study of the political leadership of Poplarism, 1919–25

Alan Johnson

Introduction

'The most effective protest of our time against the theory that the poor must be humble, contrite and respectful.' That was Harold Laski's judgement on 'Poplarism' (1928: vix), the poor people's movement led by the elected councillors and guardians in Poplar who made 'a deliberate attempt to use the existing institutions of local government ... to protect and maintain working class living standards in the ... continuous depression of the 1920's' (Ryan 1978: 56).[1] In this chapter I do not retell the story of Poplarism (see Branson 1979), but ask what lessons we can draw from the episode concerning the *making* of poor people's movements. In particular, I examine what Poplarism can tell us about the role of political leadership and strategy in the success and failure of poor people's movements and how socialist politics based on the concept of mass mobilization from below can mediate differences and construct unity between the oppressed so as to 'bind the rebels together to fight for the things that matter' as George Lansbury, the radical socialist leader of Poplar Council, put it (Schneer 1990: 123).

In the first part of the chapter I locate the *making* of Poplarism within its historical context: the political economy and social structure of Poplar, and the rise and fall of a cycle of protest which stretched from the Great Unrest of 1910–14 to the General Strike of 1926. In the second half, I make the case for a reinstatement of the contingent skills and acts of what I call *the conversation of political leadership* and *the grammar of political strategy* to the heart of how we understand poor people's movements by a thematic treatment of both as they are found in Poplarism. The argument engages critically with Fox-Piven and Cloward's seminal text, *Poor People's Movements:*

Why They Succeed, How They Fail (1977). I suggest in the conclusion that the role of leadership and strategy in such movements has been relatively neglected in social policy analysis under the influence of that text. Alongside its great merit in reinstating the role of popular revolt from below, it has also sponsored more dubious themes: a myth-cum-cult of spontaneity, an ultra-left rejection of the fight for reforms, in fact of *politics per se*, and an overly structuralist and mechanical account of the rise and fall of poor people's movements.

What was 'Poplarism'? In 1919 the newly enfranchised poor swept Labour majorities, committed to fighting poverty, to power in the Poplar Board of Guardians in April and the Poplar Borough Council in November. Poplarism began life as a term of abuse used to attack 'waste, incompetence and the giving to the poor with a lavish hand of the money of their thrifty rate-paying neighbours' (Lansbury 1933: 58) but was soon reclaimed as a badge of honour by the movement in Poplar. The conflict with the government peaked between 1921 and 1925 and ranged over three basic issues. First, the equalization of the rates across London. The maintenance of the destitute was paid from local rates so poor Poplar's rates were twice as high as rich Westminster's. And when the post-war economic crisis threw thousands on to poor relief Poplar's rates rose inexorably. As Lansbury put it, the poor were paying for the poor. To force the government to equalize the rates Poplar Council illegally refused to levy that part of the rates, some £270,000, which went to the London County Council, and the Metropolitan Police, Water and Asylum Boards. When the councillors were imprisoned for ignoring a court ruling to collect these rates a mass movement was built in their defence and a rent strike threatened. The government caved in, released the imprisoned councillors and equalized the rates in October 1921. Poplar's rates were reduced by 6s 6d in the pound while the rich of Westminster and Kensington saw their rates rise by 1s in the pound. As Edgar Lansbury, the communist son of George Lansbury and a leading Poplar councillor observed, 'Poplarism' won in weeks what 'thirty years of constitutional agitation had failed to bring about' (1933: 76). The second defining feature of 'Poplarism' was a refusal to operate the Poor Law according to deterrent principles. Poplar was surcharged by the District Auditor for paying scales of relief higher than the official government scale, ignoring 'less eligibility', and for refusing to discriminate between deserving and undeserving claimants or operate the Household Means Test. The third point of conflict between Poplar and the government was its decision to pay its employees a minimum wage of £4 per week.

The 'circumstances' of a welfare struggle

The determining conditions of Poplar's welfare struggle were a severe economic crisis which impacted upon a proletarian social structure amid a political opportunity structure defined by the rise of a cycle of protest, working-class desubordination, pauper enfranchisement and a high degree of local autonomy in the provision of relief.

The political economy and social structure of Poplarism

Economic crisis was the determining context of Poplarism. The 162,000 people of Poplar relied on the docks and associated employment in transport, haulage, railways and the manufacturing industries which clustered around the waterfront. Socially and culturally the borough was proletarian, only 2.5 per cent of the residents of Poplar were 'middle class' according to a 1928 survey. Labour was largely unskilled or casualized and irregular employment was endemic; one in four lived in poverty (Branson 1979: 12–3; Ryan 1978: 57). From mid-1920 the post-war inflationary boom collapsed, and a steep decline in foreign trade devastated employment at the docks. While Whitechapel had 0.2 outdoor paupers per thousand people, Poplar had 92.5. Unemployment Insurance soon ran out for insured workers and with no national or London-wide poor relief scheme to turn to Poplar soon faced a rates crisis *in extremis*, spending £4,600 per week in out-relief by June 1921.

The political opportunity structure of Poplarism: the rise and fall of a protest cycle

The political opportunity structure of Poplarism was defined by the rise and fall of a 'cycle of protest' (Tarrow 1989) which peaked in Britain in 1919–1920. The resulting 'desubordination' of significant layers of the working class, at a time of pauper enfranchisement and local electoral victory, utterly transformed the political significance of the limited powers held by the local elected Boards of Guardians which administered poor relief and by the borough council.

Between 1918 and 1921 Britain saw more strikes than in any other three-year period. In 1919 alone there was a general strike on the Clyde for a forty-hour week, police strikes, soldiers' mutinies and rebellion in Ireland (Rosenberg 1987). Grant and Johnson have tracked the rise and fall of a militant working-class politics during this period, at odds with moderate Labourism, marked by:

a trade unionism which united industrial action and political aims; rank and file movements, suspicious of officialdom and challenging the wartime State, the evolution of Communism and a tradition of industrial direct action and mass sympathy strikes.

(Cited in Young 1989: 15)

The East End was a stronghold of Sylvia Pankhurst's Workers Socialist Federation and on Sunday evenings a young Harry Pollitt, the future leader of the Communist party, would join her at Poplar's dock gates to argue for socialism and the Russian Revolution (Morgan 1993:16). The London Workers Committee, affiliated to the Shop Stewards and Workers Committee Movement, helped to launch the 'Hands off Russia!' campaign in January 1920 and won a great victory when dockers in London refused to coal the *S.S. Jolly Roger* with munitions for Poland. In August 1920 the Labour Party itself organized a Council of Action and threatened a general strike to stop war on Russia. Poplarism was the reflection among those reliant on poor relief of this wider desubordination of the working class as much as it was a response to the brute fact of economic crisis. Attitudes to state intervention, unemployment and poor relief among workers had been transformed by the lived experience of the trenches, by the promise of a 'land fit for heroes' and by the brief taste of full employment at the end of the war. So the working class was quick to throw off its pre-war fatalistic resignation to unemployment when the economic crisis hit in 1920 (Young 1989: 196). Vincent cites the example of the ten thousand unemployed who 'besieged the Woolwich Poor Law Union all night in an attempt to force higher scales of benefit' (1991: 60). George Lansbury had organized mass protests to the Poplar guardians until the chairman was left to plead, 'How can we discuss this matter with men standing six or seven deep behind us?' (quoted in Postgate 1951: 68). James D. Young argues that it was this preparedness of the working class to demand relief 'as a democratic right', and on a scale 'unimaginable', which rendered the Poor Law principles inoperable in the early post-war period (Young 1989: 198; Branson 1979: 82). Regularly discussed in Cabinet (Ryan 1978: 71), the protests forced the government to introduce the Out of Work Donation in 1919, the Unemployment Insurance Act in 1920 and, in effect, to urge Boards of Guardians to use a loophole in the 1911 Relief Regulation Order to grant out-relief. The depth of the crisis and the speed with which it developed – unemployment rising to a level unseen in a century in a matter of months – and the fact that many of the demonstrators were ex-soldiers further stayed the governments hand. Poplarism reflected but also stimulated the new 'desubordinated' temper of the 'poor citizen'. And this temper transformed the terms on which the contradiction between political citizenship and economic exclusion could be resolved.

It was the defeat of the General Strike in 1926 which ended the cycle of protest, although the collapse of hopes in militant direct action can be dated to the disintegration of the Triple Alliance and the subsequent defeat of the miners in 1921. Branson argues that by late 1922, 'the hope and confidence which gripped Labour supporters in 1919 had, for the most part, evaporated with the slump' (1979: 161). Poplarism was left isolated as 'the last, defiant, example of the militant spirit which had created the Council of Action in 1920' (Schneer 1990: 61), powerless to resist those government changes to poor relief in the late 1920s and early 1930s which removed welfare provision from popular pressure and separated the poor citizen from the administration of poverty. The Board of Guardians (Default) Act 1926 gave government the power to suspend Boards and appoint commissioners, powers used in West Ham, Chester-Le-Street and Bedwelty to impose a 'starvation policy'. In 1927 any guardian surcharged over £500 was now to be stopped from serving for five years under the Audit (Local Authorities) Act. The Metropolitan Common Poor Fund, the victory Poplarism had wrenched from the government in 1921, was placed under the control of Ministry of Health nominees in the Local Authorities (Emergency Provisions) Act 1928. In 1929 the government simply abolished Boards of Guardians by passing the Local Government Act and in 1934 it centralized control of relief by establishing the Unemployment Assistance Board as an agency of the central state, a response to popular pressure from below expressed through Public Assistance Committees (see Chapter 7). As Vincent notes it took 'just a decade-and-a-half of full participation by the poor in their own relief to remove the element of local responsibility which had lasted for more than three centuries' (1991: 62). The battery of Acts were 'a concentration of political power within the state in order to evade and attempt to defeat the political power of labour'. Far from democracy being the best 'shell' of capitalism the poor citizen had forced the government to ensure that 'the mechanisms of power and control [were] forced deeper into the recess of the state' (Novak 1988: 158, 156). 'Poplarism' was made impossible.

The 'making' of a welfare struggle

Poor people's movements are made by poor people with specific *capacities*. The concept of capacities refers to resources and powers possessed by collective actors understood as the outcome of their position in the regime of accumulation, which Therborn calls 'intrinsic strength', and the degree of self-consciousness and organization of the collective actor, which Therborn calls 'hegemonic capacity'. These capacities are historically and spatially variable and both materially determined and politically constructed. Class is objective and subjective, both intrinsic strength and self-identification. The concept of capacity as the outcome of both aspects of class is a useful analytical tool able to guide empirical enquiry into the conditions and dynamics of collective identity and action (Therborn 1983: 37–47). In Poplar the legacy of casualism, the divisions between different groups of workers, in particular the employed and the unemployed, and between men and women, posed problems of political mobilization and of the political mediation of difference within the poor and the poor people's movement. 'Poplarism' was the outcome of complex, contingent and creative acts which constructed political identity and action. In particular, Poplarism suggests the conversation of political leadership and the grammar of political strategy should be restored to the heart of our understanding of movements and how they can succeed.

The conversation of leadership

> the Poplar Labour movement consisted of many dedicated local so-
> cialists who were responsible for the continuous programme of educa-
> tion and organisation which gave the post-war Labour party its
> impressive grass-roots strength.
>
> (Ryan 1978: 57)

'Poplarism' was not just a spontaneous revolt of the poor but the product of socialist organizing and agitation over a long period by a political leadership organic to the Poplar working class. The mass and participatory base of the campaign was 'built by [the] consistent work' (Cliff and Gluckstein 1988: 127) of that leadership, hundreds of pioneers and propagandists of the socialist movement whose political lives had been building small branches of the Social Democratic Federation (SDF) and the Independent Labour Party (ILP), establishing trade unions against bitter employer opposition (half the jailed councillors had been lay officials in their unions), arguing for and being arrested in campaigns for Irish independence and women's suffrage. The core of the Labour group were respected socialists of various organizations, Marxists and communists among them, who came to power *late*, after long experience, gradual base-building, and involvement in working-class and community-based institutions.[2] George Lansbury said of them that they 'believed their duty was to live lives of service, teaching the masses *to think and to act for themselves*' (Lansbury 1928: 2; my italics). The élan of the Poplar Labour Group was a reflection of this 'long tradition of socialist and labour unity in the borough' (Schneer 1990: 54).

Poplarism has been misinterpreted as a mere reprise of 'a native tradition of political theatre which stretched back to the eighteenth century', and Lansbury dismissed as 'the true heir of the radical libertine John Wilkes' (Vincent 1991). While this captures the use of certain symbols and rituals of an older protest tradition it misses the fact that it was the modern traditions of socialist and trade union organizing which defined Poplarism as a modern self-controlling proletarian movement not plebeians in thrall to a showman. It was not political theatre when mass meetings of rank and file delegates of the local trade union movement were called to agree strategy before the Poplar councillors launched their defiance of the government in 1921.[3] Vincent also misses the significance of the social composition of the leadership of Poplarism. Stevedores and housewives, toolmakers and dock labourers, corn porters and railwaymen, labourers, postmen and engineers, ran the council chamber and the street protests (Branson 1979: 15; Ryan 1978: 73). This was politically important because, as James D. Young has argued, it was the social and cultural gulf between middle-class socialist intellectuals and the working class which hamstrung the socialist project in England. The elitism and condescension of the middle class, typified by the Webbs, put these intellectuals at odds with the well-springs of oppositional culture within the working class, most notably an instinctive anti-statism and anti-authoritarianism expressed, for example, in the widespread opposition to the Liberals' social policy reforms of 1906–11. Many middle-class intellectuals were hostile to what Ellen Wilkinson saw as the 'vivid, intense communal life' of the working class and the 'passionate independence' with which its indigenous institutions were maintained (cited in Young 1989: 14–15).

From the 1880s the attachment of this kind of socialist intellectual to the labour movement was one factor in the victory of a statist socialism from above. Their emotional identification with the educated middle class and their 'elitist fear of a mass popular movement' led them to crush in their embrace 'the latent forces of militant socialism-from-below' which existed within the working class (Young 1989: 33). Seeing *themselves* as the heroic subject of social change they sought only to adapt the structures of the state to integrate an object, the working class, which they viewed with a mix of fear and pity, into a new social-democratic order (see Novak 1988: 90–139). In Poplar, in sharp contrast, the absence of such social and cultural distance and the presence of a militant socialist politics made possible a process of mutual learning, in which leadership became a conversation rather than a lecture. Strategy was not the preserve of the councillors alone but emerged from their conversation with an organized mass movement capable of re-educating and radicalizing its own 'leaders'. For instance, Lansbury's earlier obsession with labour colonies (Ryan 1978: 66; Schneer 1990: 41) and willingness to use the discourse of the 'malingerer' and the 'loafer' (Ryan 1978: 59–60; Vincent 1991: 24) was replaced, under the impress of the agitation of the unemployed, by an explicit repudiation of the 1834 principles and a conscious attempt to use the power of local democracy to defend the poor. His leadership of 'Poplarism' was the result of his own life-long conversation in which the rebellious voices of suffragettes, Indian and Irish nationalists, pacifists, striking workers and Russian revolutionaries were at least as insistent as his own and from which he *learnt*. But in thousands of meetings Lansbury, and scores of agitators like him, also taught as they 'met the doubts of the half-converted [and] discussed with infinite patience the immediate problems faced by activists and workers' (Postgate 1951: 97). The conversation of leadership was also carried by the *Daily Herald* which Lansbury edited. An authority in the working class after the war, with a 330,000 circulation, the *Daily Herald* was a genuine tribune of the people, feminist, anti-imperialist and socialist. It often generalized and unified diverse struggles by drawing connections and building alliances. In the summer of 1920 it carried the news of the Russian Revolution and stimulated the 'Hands off Russia!' campaign (Wicks 1992: 28). And when the unemployed protests got going the *Herald* launched a 'Go to the Guardians' campaign, urging the unemployed to mass together and besiege the guardians until they won out-relief.

Political leadership was able to take on this conversational quality in Poplar because of the 'thoroughly democratic lines' on which the campaign was run and because the formal leaders had an organic relationship to layer after layer of leaders in the mass movement (Schneer 1990: 62). For example, in March 1921 the rates strike began only 'after a conference of representatives from trade union branches where every aspect of the proposed action had been considered' (Branson 1979: 168). When Harry Wicks observed that 'the people around Lansbury were capable of tuning into the thoughts of large sections of advanced workers' (1992: 64) it was really a comment on the mass movement as much as about Lansbury. For example, the overflowing mass meetings which punctuated the campaign were 'only the visible outcrop; beneath the surface was a confused network of communication which hummed with life'. There were seventy trade union branches in Poplar, the majority affiliated to the Trades Council and Borough Labour Party and 2,800 individual Labour Party members in South Poplar alone, their penny-a-week dues collected by activists who functioned as permanent persuaders carrying the news and arguments of the campaign. The councillors 'spent their lives in close contact with the problems of Poplar's workplaces' and many were 'the acknowledged leaders among their fellow workers on the job' or were in 'active contact' with women through the Maternity and Child Welfare Committee. The result was 'an unusually active and participating electorate [who] came to political meetings of all kinds, were stirred by what they heard, raised their voices, were drawn in and consulted and, from time to time, were filled with excitement and a sense of purpose' (Branson 1979: 167–9). As Cliff and Gluckstein argue, 'Poplar's councillors did not substitute themselves for action, they *led* it. Between 1919 and 1923 the masses were not used as a means to win council seats and then protect them. The councillors saw their role as serving the workers movement' (1988: 128).

Moreover, because the Poplar councillors were the advanced section *of* the Poplar working class they were able, unlike the middle-class intellectual socialists, to draw upon the native organizational and cultural capacities of the working class: networks of mutual aid and 'friendly leads' (street collections), hostility to 'the acquisitive individualism of capitalist society', and distrust of outside institutions and their representatives (see Young 1989: 1–16). Lansbury himself possessed a well developed contempt for the Toynbee Hall or Fabian expert, 'peeping and prying into the homes of the poor', according to his son Edgar Lansbury (1933: 158). Young argues that this class hostility to the 'expert' was a well-spring of the capacity of self-reliance. When the Poplar councillors were imprisoned in 1921 this capacity was reflected in the rise of the Tenants Defence League, a body which organized street by street for a rent strike should any attempt be made to collect the rates while the councillors were imprisoned. The League 'grew by leaps and bounds, organising rallies and distributing placards to members who then displayed them in their windows' (Schneer 1990: 58). And this too was the conversation of leadership, here borne from house to house by activist-neighbours, trusted and known, and organized into committees in every ward (Branson 1979: 92).

Finally, this conversation of leadership was continued when the Labour group negotiated with the government. While Edgar Lansbury was able to out-argue the Ministry of Health officials on the details, *politically* the leaders sought only to 'throw the voice' of the mass movement upward at the government. They reasoned the government would only give way because 'the mass is as solid as a rock'. So when the councillors were in prison they refused to negotiate until they were released and refused to purge their contempt to get released. They saw the task of leadership as sustaining the strength of the movement beyond the prison walls for they knew that was the only real power the campaign possessed. This democratic calculation led the councillors to simply 'burn their boats' during negotiations and to speak in 'plain unmistakable terms' that 'we shall not give way' (Branson 1979: 46–7).

The grammar of strategy

> The Labour Movement here had to face the question which sooner or later, nationally and locally, the whole movement will have to answer: 'You now have the power – what are you going to do with it ? ... *We have come to make a change*'.
>
> (Councillor Charles Key, 1923, quoted in Branson 1979: 162)

I have argued that the conversational character of the leadership of Poplarism was made possible because of the organic relationship between it and the base of the campaign. But it was the *strategy* adopted by the Poplar councillors which made this sociological fact into a *politically* relevant one. *The grammar of strategy structures the conversation of leadership.* Leadership is a series of purposive acts, relationships and skills (Barker, Johnson, Lavalette, forthcoming (a)) but these are inseparable from strategic questions such as how and when to act, who to ally with and for what attainable ends in light of relatively abstract conceptions of the nature of society and the possibilities for change within it (Barker, Johnson, Lavalette, forthcoming (b)).

The strategy of Poplarism was distinguished in three senses: content, form and agency. First, the *content* of the struggle was an attempt to use the local council chamber and the Board of Guardians to stimulate and lead a movement in pursuit of felt diverse working-class need regardless of any other competing rationale, legal or economic. Second, the struggle, though I acknowledge it was scarcely conscious of itself in this regard, took the *form* of a 'transitional' politics, seeking to bridge minimum reforms and maximum goal. Third, it was a politics of commonality, using discursive practice and policy to mediate difference and construct a new collective actor, 'working people', as the *agency* of change.

Content: Poplarism as a politics of need

Poplarism was a politics of human need which in 'reject[ing] the basic assumptions of the deterrent Poor Law' (Ryan 1978: 76–7) meant that the councillors were refusing to 'remain confined within the limits of the system in which they found themselves' (Branson 1979: 27). As George Lansbury explained in his autobiography:

> I took it as my policy that no widow or orphan, no sick, infirm or aged person should lack proper provision of the needs of life, and able-bodied people should get work or maintenance.
>
> (Lansbury 1928: 135)

George Lansbury famously declared that 'If we have to choose between contempt of the poor and contempt of Court, it will be contempt of Court' (quoted in Branson 1979: 46).[4] When, in August 1923, the Board of Guardians paid relief, illegally again, to dock strikers, and faced a hysterical press reaction, Edgar Lansbury said simply that the strikers 'had been able to stand up to the employers with a full belly' (Branson 1979: 190). The rates were deliberately used as a means of local wealth redistribution (only one-third of rates was paid by local residents, the rest by industrial and commercial firms). Maternity and welfare services were expanded, more health visitors appointed and free milk distributed en masse. New public baths were opened and 150 new houses were built. Slum landlords were ordered to make their properties fit for human habitation. If they failed the council did the work itself and sent the errant landlord the bill (Lansbury 1933: 241). The death rate in Poplar fell from 22.7 per 1,000 in 1918 to 11.2 per thousand in 1923 and infant mortality fell from 110 to 59 in the same period. This was 'the lowest rate for the 95 largest towns in Britain' (Cliff and Gluckstein 1988: 127).[5] The campaign pamphlet *Guilty and Proud of It: Poplar's Answer* (1922) explicitly proclaimed this politics of need to the world: 'The people of Poplar have steadily supported the view that the duty of members of the Board of Guardians is to be Guardians of the POOR and not the Guardians of the interests of property' (quoted in Branson 1979: 144). When the District Auditor quashed the £4 minimum wage Poplar paid to its council employees and surcharged the councillors for their extravagance he made clear that their real crime had been to ignore the market rate (Branson 1979: 179). And with the demand for 'work or full maintenance' the politics of need challenged not just the imperatives of profit and the role of government but the very *purposes* of production. Needs-based politics is a direct threat to the state because, as Vincent has noted, 'the more the poor were helped according to their diverse needs, the greater the danger that the state would lose the capacity to reform or punish the ever-present residuum' (1991: 24). Poplarism was an example of what Kate Soper, the socialist and feminist philosopher, has called a politics of 'true need' for it stood not just for the satisfaction of biological exigencies but it also posed the Aristotelian question, 'what is needed as a condition of human flourishing and happiness?', and as such was an 'ends-questioning' rather than just a 'means-contending' form of politics (1990: 46). Listen, for example, to Poplar Councillor Helen McKay (a trade unionist, a member of the Marxist Social Democratic Federation, arrested during the suffragette campaign), as she sits opposite Sir Alfred Mond, the Minister of Health and calmly tells him why she is going to break the law and ignore the scales of relief he has set:

> You know Sir, that down in our area we have a great deal of tubercular trouble, also in children physical conditions which develop into tubercular trouble. Whenever such a family comes under our notice, with housing conditions as they are we cannot say what we should say in a great many cases – you should get a larger house; but we can say – you must rearrange your sleeping arrangements, that will help the situation. What is going to be the result of this scale? Inevitably the result will be that a family who is already overcrowded will take in a lodger ... and they will do it against their better judgement.
>
> (Quoted in Branson 1979: 155)

Form: Poplarism as a transitional politics

By refusing to remain 'confined within the limits of the system in which they found themselves' Poplarism reached for a standard beyond bourgeois right: the standard of human need. But human need is normally considered a standard of distributive justice belonging to the future socialist society 'as it has developed on its own foundations' for 'right can never be higher than the economic structure of society and its cultural development conditioned thereby' (Marx [1875] 1969: 19). *Transitional* politics is a response to the question this begs: how do we get there? In other words, how can a collective actor be forged in *this* present capable of producing *that* future? The tradition of socialism from below has generally answered this question by pointing to the potential for the self-emancipation of the majority through a militant struggle for its needs, this struggle being, potentially at any rate, at once *educative*, stimulating a process of 'self-changing', and *instrumental*, a means for the 'changing of circumstances'. This political method can be traced back to the *Communist Manifesto* in which Marx and Engels insist that socialists 'fight for the attainment of the immediate aims, for the enforcement of the momentary interests of the working class; but in the movement of the present they also represent and take care of the future of the movement' ([1848] 1973: 97). In 1921, the very year of Poplar's rates victory, this method was developed further by the Communist or Third International in the *Theses on Tactics*, a document replete with the language of need. A militant fight for *present* needs, conducted without regard for the 'needs' of capital, argued the Comintern, can be the bridge to the *future* society. The *Theses* urged a fight for reforms focused on the needs of 'the broadest masses', for 'demands whose fulfilment is an immediate and urgent working class need'. Principles of justice which 'belong' to the future society are reached for in order to build a bridge to that society in the present. And that bridge is not pieces of legislation or the incremental growth of collectivization but the spiritual growth of a collective actor, organized, conscious, and self-controlling. Transitional politics, then, stands at the heart of Marx's conception of socialism as the self-emancipation of the working class because it is the rational political expression of the philosophical understanding of the *simultaneity* of the constitution of the emancipatory subject and the struggle for its needs, of 'the coincidence of the changing of circumstances and self-changing'. Poplarism in its use of Council chamber and Board of Guardians gives us a glimpse of what it can mean to give democratic forms a new social content. The Poplar leaders were no naïve reformists. Lansbury was clear that, 'we are not going to end Capitalism by Poplar methods'. But as Branson points out, what set Poplarism apart was its impact on the working class for it proclaimed that 'a new kind of life was possible' and so 'encourag[ed] the downtrodden to stand up' (1979: 166).

The infusion of explicitly socialist propaganda into the struggle generalized, bound together and gave a wider political meaning to each immediate struggle. The leaders of Poplarism – and it should be clear by now there were thousands of such leaders – agitated from platform and paper, leaflet and prison cell. They carried subversive ideas which reframed the struggle for the listener, as they argued that production could be organized for need not profit, that unemployment and low wages were a necessary part of capitalism, that government policy reflected the needs of capitalism, that ministers like Mond were a tool of the ruling class, that the legal system would always preserve the *status quo*, that workers should rely on nothing but their own strength. But the embedding of this discursive practice *in the institutional texture of working-class life* and in the hurdy-gurdy of political struggle mattered profoundly, for it moved people because it was received and amplified by that 'confused network of communication which hummed with life' and because it generalized the lived experience of an immediate struggle for need.[6]

Agency: Poplarism as a politics of commonality

The strategy of Poplarism in the realm of agency was, as George Lansbury put it, 'to bind all the rebels together to fight for the things that matter' (Schneer 1990: 123). The leaders were conscious that 'social policy' was a battleground on which the ruling class and the state had *constructed division*. The discourse of 'social policy' during this period, from Chamberlain on the right to the Webbs on the left, was self-consciously divisive, its very purpose being to prevent the skilled organized unemployed from 'identify[ing] their lot with that of the casual and chronic poor' (Novak 1988: 100). The battle between Poplar and the government over the level of poor relief was not just about the material living standard of the recipients. It was also a symbolic or discursive clash over the prospects for political unity between claimants and other workers. At stake was the *impact upon identity* of poor relief. The government sought to drive down the level of relief faster than cuts in wages so relief would continue to function as a deterrent and *divide* the employed worker from the unemployed worker. Poplarism sought to *unite* the unemployed and employed by establishing a discourse, embodied in policy, that no *working person* should be allowed to fall below a level set by a measure of human need. The pamphlet *Guilty and Proud of It: Poplar's Answer* (1922), accused the Poor Law of dividing 'the employed against the unemployed, the deserving against the undeserving, and the healthy against the sick' and of defining poverty as a crime and the pauper as a criminal. The pamphlet claimed that 'In Poplar there is no cringing ... Relief is accepted without shame or regret'. And when between 1921 and 1924 there was 'the sharpest fall in wages and prices known to British history' (Branson 1979: 173), Poplar refused to follow the private sector and other labour councils and reduce wages, insisting the council should maintain a minimum living standard. Once again this was not only a defence of the living standards of the council employees but a conscious political effort to help those in work to fight wage cuts and to *constitute* the collective actor, 'working people'. So when *The Times* editorial wrote that Poplar was creating 'an army of wastrels', Charlie Sumner responded, 'the fact that independent workmen are receiving inadequate wages ... is no reason for giving less relief than will properly maintain the families on public assistance ... the Guardians' opinion is that the working people are entitled to work or maintenance' (quoted in Branson 1979: 126). But this discursive battle, which Volosinov, the Russian linguist, called the 'clash of live social accents', far from floating free of any social foundation, was rooted in class experience and relations. In any welfare struggle the ruling class and government attempt to 'impart a supra-class, eternal character to the ideological sign, to extinguish or drive inward the struggle between social value judgements which occurs in it' (Volosinov, in Collins 1996: 76). Poplarism is important not just because these signs – 'wastrels' 'spendthrift', 'feckless', 'lax', 'lavish' – were *contested* in the utterances of the campaign – 'working people', 'need', 'entitlement', 'happiness', 'greedy profit monger', but also because these counter utterances were *effective in the world*. Poplarism's discursive practice, to put it in those terms, was successful because it met three conditions set out by Volosinov (1986). First, the utterances formed an 'immanent critique'. In other words they were a critical appropriation of certain ideological signs and meanings, such as 'citizenship', to point to a radical alternative, a politics of human need. Second, this re-articulation of meaning took place within and through an actual movement of protest. Third, while contestation in linguistic exchange is part and parcel of everyone's daily experience in societies defined by exploitative and oppressive social relations, Volosinov argued that a creative political leadership was required to respond 'strategically and creatively to the problems which ... people pose for themselves in the contest over alternative futures [and] helping to provide and develop the symbolic, cultural and organisational resources with which they themselves can provide answers' (quoted in Collins 1996: 86–7). Only when so contextualized – as immanent critique, borne by a protest movement, developed creatively by a political leadership – could the utterance 'working people' even begin to interpolate or 'bind together' the employed and unemployed and trump the category of the 'waster' or 'loafer'.

Poplarism also illustrated the importance of political leadership in mediating gender difference among the poor. In May 1920 Poplar set the minimum wage for all its employees, men and women, at £4 per week. Overnight this raised wages for men by 25 per cent and for women by almost 70 per cent. Though the Labour Party had passed policy in favour of equal pay for equal work in 1918 Poplar was almost alone in taking it seriously. Five Law Lords ruled the minimum wage illegal and charged Poplar with being driven by 'a feminist ambition to secure equality of the sexes'. They did not know how right they were. George Lansbury was not only 'the chief and most visible male supporter of the feminist movement in Britain' (Schneer 1990: 68) but by 1921 had a long record of bridging and binding together the socialist and feminist movements. In 1888 Lansbury organized Jane Cobden's path-breaking election campaign for the London County Council and enabled her to address striking bargebuilders, East End shop assistants and Bass-dressers trying to establish a union. When, in 1912, he exploded at the Prime Minister Asquith in the House of Commons over his treatment of suffragettes and then resigned his Bow and Bromley seat to fight a by-election on that issue, the result was one of few examples of a socialist-feminist election campaign that Britain has ever seen. He failed but it was a magnificent failure as he worked to fuse the labour movement not just with a working-class social or domestic feminism, attentive to the diverse felt needs of working women faced with poverty, sweated labour and poor housing but with a feminism which rejected the idea of 'two spheres' and insisted, argues Schneer, that 'power or the lack of it was rooted in sex as well as class'. On the latter point Lansbury's own ideas 'had undergone a revolution' as he talked to, worked with and learnt from, militant suffragette women (Schneer 1990: 125). Lansbury argued with the working class about feminism and with suffragettes about socialism – urging that women's liberation and socialism should go hand in hand.

Universalism and particularism

What implications might Poplarism bear for the contemporary social policy debate about universalism and particularism? I tentatively suggest that it tells us what a transcendence of that antinomy might look like. Benhabib (1995) has warned of the dangers of a confluence of identity politics with a politics targeted at the redistributionist welfare state in the contemporary United States. Women, she argues, are being pitted against other groups for jobs, housing, educational opportunities and health care benefits. This competition for scarce resources has produced 'group particularisms, often with antagonistic consequences'. Despairing of the 'Balkanization of urban America' which this particularistic politics is producing, Benhabib has called for 'a new politics of civility and solidarity, robust enough in its vision to unite those social forces torn now by fragmentation and factionalism' and has urged a shift from 'the logic of redistribution to the ethics of solidarity' to enlarge mentalities until the achievement of 'a new synthesis of collective solidarities with plurally constituted identities' (1995: 36–9). In similar vein Todd Gitlin has warned that the current obsession with difference is marginalizing that 'frame of understanding and reference that understands "difference" against the background of what is not different, what is shared among groups' and has called for a new 'politics of commonality' (1994: 144).

Poplarism helps us imagine how such a politics might be created beginning with a rejection of the post-structuralist and postmodern notion that a politics of commonality 'cannot appeal to anything in the social order that would operate as its ground' (Laclau 1994: 4). For discursive practice, as we have seen, did not float free of any 'social ground' in Poplar. It was a politics of human need which facilitated a politics of commonality aimed at 'binding all the rebels together'. This suggests that human need might be the social ground of a universalism which, far from resulting in a 'disrespect for all forms of particularism' as Laclau fears, could be the ground on which all the diverse needs, all the 'sensuous particularity' as Eagleton puts it (1996: 118), can be rearticulated within a wider politics of commonality. In contrast, particularistic social policy is inescapably divisive not because it accepts the reality of diverse needs but because, in essentializing each group or identity and positioning each in a unilateral relationship to the state as a client it detaches social policy from any ethic of solidarity and therefore from any possibility of systemic social change, and so risks replicating rather than rupturing the ugly and unequal textures of capitalist society. Poplar suggests a militant fight for universalist social policy reforms sensitive to the diverse needs of the poor has the potential to be the social ground upon which unity can be constructed and difference mediated, particularism embraced but located within a wider coalition of concern.[7]

Conclusion

I conclude by reflecting on the implications Poplarism might bear for our understanding of the political making of poor people's movements. I suggest that the pivotal role of the conversation of leadership and the grammar of strategy in the making of Poplarism constitutes a challenge to the model of how poor people's movements succeed and why they fail found in Fox-Piven and Cloward's *Poor People's Movements*. I do not claim one small episode of collective action can overturn that model but I do claim it raises a series of challenging questions which might stimulate and guide future discussion about poor people's movements and collective action more generally.

The Fox-Piven/Cloward model (1977: ix–37) can be summarized thus: elites only respond to the threat of popular insurgency. The poor win when they refuse to abide by 'the norms of the electoral-representative system' and are instead *turbulent*. If, at those rare moments when the regulatory capacity of society is weakened (docility is enforced and protest structurally precluded normally) the poor engage in mass defiance and disrupt social institutions, by street protests and riots, then they can win concessions, especially if the 'calculus of electoral instability favours the protesters'. The turbulence will subside, however, and the movement will be incorporated. The concessions will be clawed back by the state unless it functions to benefit the system as a whole. Fox-Piven and Cloward, incredibly, offer the Congress of Industrial Organisations (CIO) as an example, arguing that it was not disbanded by the ruling class in the United States because 'labour unions constituted a useful mechanism to regulate the labour force'.

Any attempt by a political leadership to intervene in this process is futile and dangerous. *Futile*: leaders can call on a movement to pursue one strategy or another but this will have no effect as 'social conditions preclude the exercise of such options'. Leaders can not create protest, or shape its form, or shape the responses of elites. The organizations leaders build do not influence anything and can not prevent the inevitable ebbing of protest. Protest is determined 'by institutional conditions and not by the purposive efforts of leaders and organizers'. *And dangerous*: leaders will prioritize the development of the organization rather than the turbulence which alone will wrench concessions from the state and will 'channel the insurgent masses into normal politics' from which nothing can be gained.

Poplarism challenges this model in numerous ways. Where Fox-Piven and Cloward allow only spontaneity here was plan and leadership, where they allow only riot here was organized struggle, where they allow only for the structural determination of protest here was a dialectic of imposed necessity and cultivated desire. While they define the entire 'electoral-representative system' as an ideological trap to be avoided, here was a use of local government to advance a militant fight for reforms. Where they seem resigned to the separation of unemployed from employed the Poplar socialists strove to build an alliance between both. We can also say that a series of counter-positions found in the Fox-Piven and Cloward model seem like false antinomies in the light of Poplarism. They flatly counterpose 'mass-based permanent organisation' to 'popular insurgency' but Poplarism reminds us of the role of permanent organization in stimulating popular energies and sustaining them over a long haul. They counterpose 'workers erupting in strikes' to 'collecting dues cards' but this does little to explain the role of those dense networks of socialist and trade union organization in Poplar, built up over decades by the small labours of thousands, which formed a political and cultural resource which enhanced the 'eruption' when it came. And, rather than counterposing 'the streets' to the 'meeting rooms', as Fox-Piven and Cloward do, Poplarism suggests a political force can be he-gemonic in each because it was hegemonic in both.

Poplarism also challenges the account of agency which underpins the Fox-Piven and Cloward model. To insist that poor people's movements can only ever win as 'a response to their turbulence and not their organised numbers' is to fail to grasp that when the modern organized working class is a significant social presence the very potentialities and dynamics of popular protest are transformed. To argue it is 'inchoate anxieties and diffuse anger that drives the masses' is to bracket out the capacity – in part politically formed as we have seen – for creative self-controlling agency on the part of the modern working class, which is able to be not only angry but also self-aware and strategic. And while Fox-Piven and Cloward correctly argue that poor people, like anyone else, only protest when the target is perceived as both unjust and mutable, they never allow these moments of perception to result from processes internal to the working class but only from external factors such as the scale of the distress or the happenstance that one wing of the ruling class will enlist the lower-orders as an aid against another rival wing and then lose control. Missing again is a sense of the rich internal political life of the working class itself. Protest – in their timeless model – is simply delivered up by the contradictions of capitalism only to inevitably fail because, and this is the real premise of *Poor People's Movements*, the poor cannot control their own organizations. The model invests all real human agency – bar elemental upsurges, naturalistically conceived and doomed to fail – in the state and the bourgeoisie.

Poplarism tells us that the modern working class has the capacity to mount not just periodic 'outbursts of desperation and vengeance' but to sustain self-controlling organized 'political struggle', to use the contrasting terms with which Lenin discussed the question. There is without doubt much in the Fox-Piven and Cloward model which does illuminate the Poplar experience. In fact, as a mass rebellious upsurge from below which refused to play by the rules and which disrupted the normal functioning of the state to win concessions only for those concessions to be largely lost once the turbulence subsided Poplarism was a poor people's movement right out of *Poor People's Movements*, and reminds us of the continuing value of the book. As George Lansbury said, 'nobody bothers about the poor except when the poor commence to kick' (in Schneer 1990: 97). But Lansbury was always too modest. We need to bring back in purposive political leadership and political strategy, and capacities of creative agency, and we need to examine more closely the relationship between the two and the role of both in shaping the success and failure of poor people's movements. We need to create the space for a politics which can go beyond the poor kicking out. We need a politics that can 'bind all the rebels together to fight for the things that matter'.

Notes

1 I would like to thank Michael Lavalette, Paul Reynolds and Debbie Williams for helpful discussions about Poplarism.
2 The importance of the deep local roots and long political experience of the Poplar councillors is seen by a comparison to the fortunes of the young and inexperienced Socialist Party in the United States which took municipal power in many areas in the pre-First World War era, 'before strategies had been prepared or stable bases of support developed', and consequently found itself 'suffocated … politically before it could gain a foothold' by 'urban elites, using traditional community institutions' (Judd 1989: 15, 18).
3 Vincent's charge that the imprisoned councillors 'did everything possible to distance themselves from the common criminal' (1991: 60) is unsupported by any evidence and demands a response. Nellie Cressall was heavily pregnant when she was thrown in Holloway Prison, left for twenty-four hours alone in her cell with 'the dreadful screaming of the poor women in the padded cells' around her. George Lansbury, then an elderly man, was threatened with physical violence by warders until the screams of solidarity from his comrades stopped a beating. In fact, the councillors were initially subjected to a worse prison regime than many 'common criminals' until protests forced a change. Prison was probably responsible for the deaths soon after release of Charlie Sumner and

Minnie Lansbury. When conditions improved George Lansbury addressed a meeting of prisoners with the Governor present and said 'These people should have the same privileges as us' (Postgate 1951: 218). On release the councillors issued public statements railing against 'these modern Bastilles' and Nellie Cressall gave public talks on the conditions of women prisoners in Holloway.

4   The banner of the Liverpool Labour councillors during their conflict with the government in 1984–5 carried the words, 'Better to break the law than break the poor' seeking to draw upon the legacy of Poplarism. For a detailed account of the politics of the Militant Tendency in Liverpool at this time see Johnson (1996).

5   In contrast, George Lansbury believed he could see the results of the Mond and Chamberlain periods at the Ministry of Health, in any playground or street: the two 'bad crops' of 'stunted and diseased children, as obvious as faults in geological strata' (Postgate 1951: 241).

6   If we measure the success of Poplar in electoral terms the results are no less impressive. In 1922, while the Labour Party in London lost 300 seats and control of six councils and while in Herbert Morrison's own borough of Hackney every single Labour councillor lost, the Labour vote in Poplar went up on a larger poll. By 1924 Poplar was the safest Labour area in the country (Schneer 1990: 64).

7   For a more detailed discussion of the relationship of a politics of need to the mediation of difference and construction of a politics of commonality see, A. Johnson (forthcoming).

7 The 'two souls of socialism'

The labour movement and unemployment during the 1920s and 1930s

Laura Penketh and Alan Pratt

Introduction

In this chapter we do not intend to look solely at the struggle of the unemployed during the inter-war years. The history of the hunger marches, riots and various campaigns against the scourge of mass unemployment are already well established in the works of, for example, Branson and Heinemann (1973), Kingsford (1982) and Croucher (1987). Instead, our intention is to look at the different goals and strategies, in short the politics, of the two competing and dominant labour movement campaigns against unemployment during the 1920s and 1930s. First, there was the politics of labourism or reformism. In these years the Labour Party became a truly mass working-class party. Within its ranks were a range of individuals from the right-wing of social democracy through to revolutionary socialists, and this 'broad church' adopted a range of policy statements on poverty, unemployment and socialism. This period also witnessed the first Labour governments, the minority administrations of 1924 and 1929–31. Labour was elected on both occasions to protect the poor and oppressed, yet in government the 'class' dimension to their politics was deprioritized to one of 'national renewal and recovery' in which the interests of British capital dominated. Second, there were the various campaigns of the National Unemployed Workers Movement (NUWM). The NUWM was a Communist-led organization of the unemployed whose aims were structured around three broad objectives: the material improvement of employed and unemployed workers in the face of capitalist crisis; an attempt to overcome divisions within the working class (which the government's economic and social policy attempted to create and reinforce), and to unite employed and unemployed men and women in the militant struggle for reform. In this sense the activities of the NUWM were not simply intended to highlight the blight of unemployment, but were to emphasize the fact that unemployment and the attack on workers' conditions was an inevitable consequence of capitalism in crisis.

Using Draper (1996), the fundamental difference in these approaches is between 'socialism from above' and 'socialism from below': the two souls of socialism. 'Socialism from above' is something to be imposed on the majority from above by an enlightened minority, and which:

> concentrates social-democratic attention on the parliamentary super-structure of society and on the manipulation of the 'commanding heights' of the economy ... which makes them hostile to mass action from below.
>
> (Draper 1996: 5)

By contrast, 'socialism from below' is based on the principle of the self-emancipation of the masses struggling to take charge of their own destiny and which attempts to win people to this goal via a 'transitional politics', aimed at convincing increasing numbers of workers – by argument and in practice – that meeting human need is incompatible with capitalism. Thus within the two conceptions of socialism we witness two radically different goals and leading from this different strategies for dealing with political questions in any particular period.

In what follows, we start by outlining the context within which these competing strategies unfold in the 1920s and 1930s, we then look at the dominant state discourse on economic and social policy, and, finally, we examine in more detail the two approaches for dealing with mass unemployment.

Unemployment in the 1920s and 1930s

Our understanding of the economic history of Britain between 1919 and 1939, especially the economic history of the 1930s, has been changed in some important ways by much of the historical research of the last twenty years (Stevenson and Cook 1977). However, even this 'revisionist' history cannot alter the fact that unemployment of the insured population never fell below Pigou's 'intractable' million. Because of the exclusion of certain occupations from the unemployment insurance scheme for much of this period (for example, domestic servants, agricultural workers, teachers), and the failure to register those under the age of 16 and most women, the actual numbers of unemployed and available for work were much higher than official figures allowed. Even so, registered unemployment reached a peak in 1932 of 2,828 million, 22 per cent of the insured workforce (Whiteside 1991: 2) and from 1921–39 unemployment averaged 14.7 per cent (Gray 1985).

These, of course, are national figures and give no indication of the enormous variations that existed between the regions in what was an economy experiencing profound change. One of the most important aspects of the 'revisionist' history alluded to above is its success in reminding us of the growth of new industries in the Midlands and Greater London which because of the development of a national system of electricity supply were freed from the necessity of locating near to traditional sources of power and therefore could position themselves closer to the growing market for products such as motor cars, cycles, chemicals, and electrically-powered consumer items. For workers employed in these industries real income increased, not least because of stable or falling prices.

In contrast, millions of people in the working-class communities of the old industrial heartlands, where the staple industries of coal, cotton textiles, heavy engineering and shipbuilding were concentrated, had their lives blighted by long-term unemployment and by govern-ment policies directed to the relief of unemployment. Throughout the inter-war period, and not just in the 1930s, men, women and children in central Scotland, Northern Ireland, South Wales and the north of England were faced with a bewildering series of changes in unemploy-ment assistance and unemployment insurance programmes.

These developments drastically altered the structure and balance of the main communities in Britain, leading to large-scale migration to the south-east in particular, for example:

> From ... 1931 to 1938 alone, the population of Greater London increased by nearly half a million, while that of Northumberland and Durham fell by thirty-nine thousand and that of South Wales by one hundred and fifteen thousand.
>
> (Branson and Heinemann 1973: 61)

The goals of state economic policy

Faced with this situation, what was the response of the government and the state? Conventional wisdom has it that the unemployed acquiesced in their unemployment, it was an act of God not susceptible to politically driven attempts to challenge it. Consequently, whenever working-class discontent emerged it was, allegedly, directed not against the fact of unemployment but at the attempts made by government at both central and local levels to drive down the cost of unemployment benefit to a more acceptable and affordable level and, as part of this process, to tighten up regulations governing eligibility to and administration of these benefits. This chapter explores some aspects of working-class resistance to the policies operationalized by successive governments throughout the period in respect of the continuing high levels of unemployment which orthodox classical economic theory said could not exist.

Classical political economy had no problems with the existence of frictional, structural and cyclical unemployment, indeed they were the natural and normal characteristics of a free-market capitalist economy and their solution (if any were required) could be left to market mechanisms with, perhaps, a little intervention from the state through such agencies as employment exchanges which might encourage that 'organized fluidity of labour' of which Beveridge was so fond. Voluntary unemployment likewise, could be easily dealt with by the denial of benefit. What classical economic theory could not countenance was involuntary unemployment, people being without jobs because there were no jobs to do. Say's Law guaranteed that there would always be some job available for any willing worker provided that the labour market, as an integral part of the wider market economy, was allowed to operate in a full and unhindered way. If any such worker could not find a job then it was because there were institutional forces in operation preventing the labour market from achieving its optimal allocative efficiency (for a recent, brief discussion of the work of Jean Baptiste Say, see Callinicos 1999: 229–30). For ruling-class intellectuals, politicians and policy-makers alike the most obvious candidate for blame was the trade union movement which used its collective bargaining power to prevent the movement of wages downward by an amount sufficient to make it worthwhile for employers to take more labour. Marginal cost had to equal marginal price and by keeping wages higher than market conditions warranted the unions were pricing their members out of work.

Classical political economy found a natural and receptive home in the Treasury and throughout the inter-war years it remained the dominant intellectual and policy paradigm, successfully resisting all challenges from competing non-socialist visions (it goes without saying that socialist ideas never got a look in). What these competing explanations lacked was a theory with at least equivalent explanatory power and sophistication, and this only became available with the publication of Keynes' *General Theory* in 1936. The 'Treasury view' remained dominant and it was only in the very different circumstances of total war which obtained from the spring of 1940 that attitudes changed. Even then the significance of this change of attitudes to Keynes' ideas has been fiercely debated by historians (MacLeod 1983). Britain remained the only significant capitalist nation in the 1930s not to engage in deficit financing, except for what was to be a time-limited rearmament budget.

Although Keynes demonstrated that full employment was a special and not a general case (which Say's Law had asserted) his earlier work had much in common with more orthodox economic theory. Like his fellow economists Keynes had believed that excessive real wages was the particular problem afflicting the old staple industries where long-term involuntary unemployment was concentrated (MacLeod 1983). These staple industries were also heavily involved in international trade and if their fortunes were to be revived they would have to regain their international competitiveness and become more resistant to the penetration of domestic markets by foreign competitors. How, then, to drive down real wages, especially in industries in which there was a high degree of trade union organization?

The main economic policy objective of British governments after the First World War was to return to the *status quo ante bellum*. The war had done enormous damage to Britain's patterns of trade, old markets had been lost and the domestic market penetrated to some extent at least. It must also be remembered that unlike every other major economy, Britain remained committed to free trade until 1932. To the Treasury, cuts in real wages seemed the most sensible and intellectually defensible means of restoring lost competitiveness, market share and full employment to the export oriented staple industries. This was the real reason for the return to the Gold Standard at pre-1914 parity with the dollar in 1925. Although this decision massively over-priced British exports and thus risked further job losses, workers were supposed to recognize the new reality and price themselves back into work by accepting lower money (and real) wages.

The direction of state social policy in the crisis years

In the context of economic crisis we can identify two dominant trends in state social policy objectives. First, there is a clear strategy to cut benefits, reinforce 'less eligibility' and use this as a mechanism to force down wages – social policy as a tool of the dominant economic policy paradigm. This approach raises the question of the relationship between income from employment, especially low paid employment, and income from state benefits. If workers in the export staples were to price themselves back into work then less eligibility had to be restored and the level of unemployment benefit reduced in money (and real) terms so that the new, lower wages in textiles, iron and steel, mining, etc., would become 'more eligible' than hitherto. The restoration of work incentives through a more overt application of less eligibility and the re-imposition of the disciplinary characteristics of the benefit system via a tightening up of administrative procedures and eligibility criteria were to become vital instruments of policy, especially after 1931, as successive governments sought to reduce unemployment according to the nostrums of classical political economy.

Second, a number of factors develop to promote a more interventionist state social policy. Among the most important here is the response to the substantial wave of working-class protest in the post-war era (which only fully recedes with the defeat of the General Strike in 1926) which led some commentators to argue tentatively for a mild corporatism and incorporation of layers of the trade union and labour movement bureaucracy. Middlemas (1979) suggests that sections of the British political elite identified the search for stability as the overarching objective of public policy, a stability to be achieved by the adoption of 'corporate bias'. Stability was impossible without the willing co-operation of business and labour and it is in the 1920s that we can see the birth of that process which led to the development of formal institutions and instruments characteristic of economic and social policy during the period of the 'classic welfare state' of the 1950s and 1960s.

The demands of the newly expanding industries and the needs of an advanced economy also promoted different social policy strategies: social policy as mere social control did not match the long-term economic and political goals of sections of British capital. Finally, the move towards an increasingly centralized state social policy administration was in part a reaction against local pressures brought to bear on Poor Law guardians by working-class activists.

These conflicting objectives present us with an important contradiction. As we have seen, the imperatives of economic policy demanded something like the reimposition of the post-1834 Poor Law while the search for domestic stability suggested a more conciliatory stance. How, if at all, was this contradiction resolved? In essence it never was resolved. What happened throughout the 1920s and 1930s was a series of events and outcomes which reflected judgements by policy-makers about the balance of power at critical times between capital and labour. By the end of the First World War organized labour was in a powerful position, not least because of the full employment generated by the war. In 1920 nearly 50 per cent of the labour force belonged to a union and collective bargaining had become more widespread. For Whiteside,

> the emergence of the labour movement as a major political force did more than anything else to change the whole framework within which unemployment was framed and discussed. It was no longer politically feasible to talk in terms of an impartial, 'scientific' solution to labour market problems.
>
> (Whiteside 1991: 70)

The strength of the labour movement, together with fears about the examples provided by the revolutions in Russia, Germany and elsewhere in Europe, encouraged Lloyd George's government to abandon the strict actuarial principles of the unemployment insurance scheme and to introduce at the end of the war an 'out of work donation' for servicemen and civilians alike which provided non-discriminatory unemployment benefit 'virtually on demand and at roughly four times the pre-war rate'. This scheme was abolished some two years afterward in the rapidly rising unemployment of the winter of 1920–1, but a precedent had been established and over the next ten years a series of temporary measures provided state help outside the Poor Law to those who had no statutory right to claim it (Whiteside 1991: 74–5). A significant factor in this series of pragmatic policy adjustments was the government's persistent fear about what the unemployed might do if it ever attempted to impose a social policy gospel entirely in accord with classical political economy.

The balance of power shifted in the second half of the 1920s, a shift symbolized by the retreat of the Trades Union Congress (TUC) in the General Strike and the defeat of the miners after a long and bitter struggle in 1926. The Wall Street Crash in October 1929 led to the collapse of the German and other European economies whose recovery had been based on financial credits from the United States and a more general decline in world trade soon followed. In 1931 the second Labour government fell as a consequence of the financial crisis which engulfed it and one result of this harsher environment was a significant hardening in public policy, especially towards the unemployed.

The formation of a National government headed by Ramsay MacDonald in 1931 was soon followed by a 10 per cent cut in benefit levels and the restoration of the insurance scheme to an actuarial basis. Those of the unemployed who had exhausted their right to unemployment benefit were put on transitional payments (see above) administered by local Public Assistance Committees (PACs) which had been given responsibility for the administration of unemployment assistance following the abolition of the Poor Law Boards of Guardians in the Local Government Act 1929. In 1934 the system was changed once more and the long-term unemployed became the responsibility of the Unemployment Assistance Board (UAB). Married women had their right to benefit cut as did other non-household heads, a development particularly damaging for young people. Whiteside's grim judgement of the nature of these changes is exactly right:

> It ... represent[ed] the final demise of the ... demand for subsistence level benefits available as of right to all in search of work ... under the reforms introduced in 1931 and 1934 long-term claimants were returned to less eligibility and the household means test
>
> (Whiteside 1991: 80)

The fact that much of the anger which these changes provoked was directed at the local rate reminds us of the continuing importance of the local administration of social provision. Throughout the 1920s the labour movement had been much more successful in the localities than it had been in challenging and changing national policy. Legislation in 1918 had extended the right to vote to all men over 21 and to women over 30. Moreover, it also provided for the abolition of pauper disqualification. As a consequence of those new electoral realities many Labour controlled authorities and Boards of Guardians not only provided limited public works programmes for the unemployed but also levels of poor relief in excess of permitted levels.

Inevitably these political arrangements produced wide variations in practice at local level. For example, an official survey in 1933 showed that in response to a question about how they would assess ten specimen cases, West Ham PAC arrived at a figure of £12.55 for total assistance while Blackpool offered only £3.63, Rotherham offered the full rate of assistance in 98 per cent of cases but in Birmingham 35 per cent were disallowed (Whiteside 1991: 81–2). What the Treasury regarded as over-generous provision was one of the reasons why the UAB was created in 1934. The UAB's attempt to impose national scale rates for the long-term unemployed helped claimants in Lancashire and East Scotland but penalized people elsewhere, especially in North East England and South Wales. The result was an explosion of anger which forced the government to introduce the 'Standstill Order' which allowed for the payment of the higher of the local PAC's rate or the national scale rates (Ryan 1981). Against this background how did the Labour Governments respond?

'Socialism from above' – the response of the Labour Party leadership

In 1924 and 1929–31 Britain witnessed the first two Labour administrations, albeit minority ones, to be elected on a platform of welfare expansion and protecting the poor, and, as noted above, there were trends within the state bureaucracy which seemed to advocate a more interventionist and expansive welfare settlement. Although the economy, especially after 1929, did face severe crisis there were nevertheless, as discussed earlier, pockets of economic expansion, and as Miliband (1972) notes, Britain had one of the richest ruling classes in the world. In this context, what actions did Labour take to advance and protect the living standards of the poor and disadvantaged? After all, the rationale of parliamentary political parties is that they will be elected to power, to govern, to direct state and society in the direction they want it to go.

At the end of the First World War the Labour Party was, in essence, recreated as a mass party of the working class. The 1918 Constitution containing the 'old' Clause IV was passed and a policy document *Labour and the New Social Order* argued the need for society as a whole to be reconstructed, to include nationalization of some of the 'commanding heights' of the economy, progressive taxation and an expansion of welfare provision. These policies were not 'revolutionary' in the sense of fundamentally challenging the dominant social relations, but were a 'blue print for a more advanced, more regulated form of capitalism' (Miliband 1972: 62). Nevertheless, many socialist activists joined the Labour Party in the hope that a future Labour government would represent real and significant change. Such activists were to play a very important and crucial role in a range of struggles over the next two decades: the unemployed movement, the General Strike, the struggle against fascism, support for the republicans in the Spanish Revolution, but many of their hopes and aspirations were to be quashed by the activities of the Labour Party leadership.

When Labour was elected in 1924 its supporters believed that the new Cabinet symbolized a working-class capture of the state. However, consequent developments revealed that Labour underwent an important qualitative change when elected, and that a new relationship was about to emerge between the Labour Party, the ruling class and the working class. The right-wing thrust of the new government was established early on when MacDonald compiled a list of potential Cabinet representatives dominated by the Labour right. He then told the opening session of the new parliament:

> We shall concentrate not first of all on the relief of unemployment, but on the restoration of trade ... and the necessity of expenditure ... will be judged in relation to the greater necessity for maintaining undisturbed the ordinary financial facilities.
>
> (*Hansard* 12 February 1924)

Philip Snowden at the Exchequer had, in opposition, favoured heavy direct taxation to redistribute wealth to the poor. However, when in office he described his role as follows:

> It is not part of my job ... to put before the House of Commons proposals for the expenditure of public money. The function of the Chancellor of the Exchequer, as I understand it, is to resist all demands for expenditure made by his colleagues and, when he can no longer resist, to limit the concession to the barest point of acceptance.
>
> (Cited in Cliff and Gluckstein 1988: 101)

The mildly favourable economic circumstances meant that Labour could afford to offer certain welfare reforms such as grants to schools and slight increases to benefits via the Unemployed Insurance Acts. However, these were only marginally different from what the openly pro-capitalist parties could have done in similar circumstances. The partial economic recovery also led workers to believe that they could, with the election of a Labour government, achieve some improvements in their working conditions. They were to be proved wrong as after a spate of strikes following Labour's victory the Cabinet set in motion the 'blacklegs charter', the Emergency Powers Act, which included strike-breaking provisions. Although this was difficult for the unions to accept, their loyalty to the Labour Party meant they felt compelled to implement the government's ruling, and they were instrumental in imposing a settlement. This was part of MacDonald's attempts to prove Labour's worth to the ruling class and stress its respectable credentials. Trotsky's analysis of the Labour leadership during this period was blistering. He stated:

> The vulgarly optimistic Victorian epoch, when it seemed that tomorrow would be a little better than today and the day after that a bit better than tomorrow, has found its most finished expression in the Webbs, Snowden, MacDonald and the other Fabians. ... These pompous authorities, pedants and haughty highfalutin' cowards are systematically poisoning the labour movement, clouding the consciousness of the proletariat and paralysing its will. It is only thanks to them that Toryism, Liberalism, the Church, the monarchy, the aristocracy and the bourgeoisie continue to survive. ... The Fabians, the ILP'ers and the conservative trade union bureaucrats today represent the most counterrevolutionary force in Great Britain, and possibly in the present stage of development, in the whole world. ... Workers must at all costs be shown these ... liveried footmen of the bourgeoisie in their true colours.
>
> (Trotsky 1974 [1925]: 57)

The second Labour-led administration was elected in 1929, with the promise that its goal was to tackle unemployment and improve the lot of the unemployed. MacDonald prophesied: 'I have reason to believe that this Government will go down into history as the Government of Employment' (*Daily Herald*, 17 June 1929). At the Labour Conference in 1930 he argued:

> [Capitalism] has broken down, not only in this little island. It has broken down in Europe, in Asia, in America: it has broken down everywhere. ... And the cure ... the new path, the new idea is organisation – organisation which will protect life, not property.
>
> (Quoted in Miliband 1972: 160)

However, the capitalist crisis led to an inexorable rise in unemployment, and by the end of 1929 the government was freely admitting that curing capitalism would be at the expense of the unemployed 'in the national interest'. When Labour came into office unemployment stood at 1.3 million, or 10 per cent of the workforce, and in its election manifesto it offered an 'unqualified pledge to deal immediately and practically with this question' (quoted in Miliband 1972: 162). But after a year in government, unemployment had risen to 2 million, and when Labour left office it was 2.7 million, or 22 per cent of the workforce (Cliff and Gluckstein, 1988: 153). Government attempts to deal with the crisis by establishing, for example, job creation schemes, were limited because the Cabinet had decided that

> we must not be rushed into shovelling out public money merely for the purpose of taking ... people off the unemployed register. ... Both for political and financial reasons, we must do all we can to combat the present feeling of insecurity in our financial prospects, and we must, therefore, avoid all schemes involving heavy additions to Budget charges or grandiose loan expenditure.
>
> (Cab.26(30), 8 May 1930, cited in Cliff and Gluckstein 1988: 153)

The record of the second Labour administration is another example of its unwillingness to fight for working-class interests while in power. Instead of honouring pre-election pledges concerned with representing and fighting for the interests of the working class, it resorted to implementing policies which were to the detriment of the poorest sections of society. Indeed, the Tory MP, Robert Boothby stated: 'It may be one of fate's little ironies that the principal task confronting the present so-called Socialist administration should be to make Great Britain safe for the capitalist' (*Hansard* 4 July 1929). Labour's attitude to the unemployed had been one of 'work or maintenance' since the days of Keir Hardie, with the assumption that if work was unavailable some degree of comfort must be provided. However, in 1931 Snowden, the Labour Chancellor of the Exchequer, told the House of Commons that drastic and disagreeable measures would have to be taken. The prime minister was to meet unions and employers to discuss employers' demands for a cut of one-third in unemployment benefit, as well as reductions in civil service pay and social services (*Daily Herald*, 17 February 1931). In May 1931 it was stated that government finances were tottering on the brink of disaster, and that in order to make savings, the dole was to be reduced by 20 per cent. Savings would have to come through the means test, with the result that benefits were withheld until claimants could prove that they had literally nothing to live on, and workers' National Insurance contributions would be raised. It was the TUC alone that prevented a complete capitulation to Labour's economy measures.

In the face of the crisis the Labour Cabinet went to the Tories and the Liberals, and asked whether a 10 per cent cut in the dole would satisfy them, and were advised to discuss this with the bankers. Labour then turned to the Bank of England and asked them 'whether', as MacDonald later told Parliament, 'in their opinion the scheme proposed would produce a loan'. Miliband continues:

> They [the bankers] thought it might and, in their turn, said they would make inquiries in New York. What this sordid tale suggests is that the Labour Government had surrendered all freedom of initiative to the Opposition leaders, to the Treasury officials, and, finally, to the goodwill of American finance.
>
> (Miliband 1972: 175)

The outcome revealed the irrelevance of elections, manifestos and promises regarding unemployment. There were demands for an immediate and swingeing attack on the most disadvantaged in society, accompanied by the condition that, should political dissent arise, then harder-line politicians would have to move in. The Cabinet voted by some 11 or 12 votes to 8 or 9 (the size of the majority is disputed), in favour of cutting unemployment benefit by 10 per cent. A narrow majority was, however, not enough for the bankers, who made it clear that the government in its entirety must join in. MacDonald failed to secure this unanimity, and ended the Labour government there and then, forming the National government with the Tories and the Liberals (Cliff and Gluckstein 1988).

In October 1931 the Labour Party lost power, and their number of seats in Parliament fell drastically from 288 to 52. The historian John Saville believes that this had serious implications for the future activities of the Labour Party. The focus on parliamentary democracy was to be intensified, and every campaign and policy proposal was to be carefully scrutinised to ensure its effectiveness in securing a Commons majority. This led to increasing attacks on internal debate within the Labour Party, and the further marginalization of working-class struggle. Miliband summarized the politics of the second Labour government thus:

> On the one hand [the Labour Party] resolutely set its face against any concessions to the Labour left. On the other, it consistently sought the co-operation and goodwill of its Conservative and particularly its Liberal opponents. Nor is this surprising. MacDonald and some of his more influential colleagues found it much easier to agree on crucial aspects of policy with Liberals and even with Conservatives than with Socialists.
>
> (Miliband 1972: 160)

Following the 1931 defeat there was an apparent radicalization within the Labour Party. This was not unusual: when Labour is thrown out of power it tends to revert to left-wing politics to appease its supporters, whereas in office it prioritizes the interests of capitalism. For example, Herbert Morrison, a right-wing Labour politician, claimed that:

> Labour must move to the Left ... to the real Socialist Left. Not the spurious left policy of handing out public money under the impression that we are achieving a redistribution of wealth under the capitalist system. That is one of the illusions of reformism.
>
> (Quoted in Cliff and Gluckstein 1988: 167)

And Hugh Gaitskell spoke of smashing the economic power of the upper class.

However, by the middle of the decade, the panic engendered in 1931 began to subside, and Empire cushioned British capital from the worst rigours of the slump. Bourgeois democracy survived, and within the Labour Party the right reasserted its dominance at the 1934 Labour Party Conference. From 1934 onwards, the labour movement, which had been dealt a devastating blow by the defeat of the 1926 General Strike and had hit a low point from 1929 to 1933, began to revive. The number of trade unionists rose from 4,392,000 in 1933 to 6,298,000 in 1939, and the number of strikes rose from 359 in 1933 to a pre-war peak of 1,129 in 1937 (Cliff and Gluckstein 1988: 173). In 1937 there were two strike waves of engineering apprentices which spread through the North and down to London and the same pattern was repeated in mining, when miners fought the breakaway union run by George Spencer. The Communist Party played a prominent part in these activities, but the Labour Party leadership only approved of moves that assisted parliamentary opposition.

This brief review of the two minority Labour administrations reveals that there were clearly things that the Labour Party could have done to stand up for and represent the poor and the oppressed in the face of capitalist crisis, at a time when even sections of the state bureaucracy were arguing for a more 'humanitarian' approach. However, in both periods Labour's priority was to run the economy on capital's terms which meant accepting the dominant bourgeois economic paradigm of the era: accepting the legitimacy of the 'Treasury view'. This involved a strategy whereby the crisis of British capitalism would be cured by increasing the rate of exploitation of workers, cutting benefits, reinforcing less eligibility, and using these as a mechanism to drive down wages. Rather than challenge such a perspective, or even follow Labour conference resolutions and commitments to 'pump prime' the economy (Miliband 1972: 163), the Labour leadership was concerned to emphasize to the dominant class its suitability for government, its respectability and its financial rectitude.

'Socialism from below' – the role of the NUWM

In the face of rising unemployment and the gradual abandonment by the leadership of the Labour Party of pursuing working-class interests, unemployed activists began to organize to fight back against attacks on their living standards. Thus, in spite of Labour's failure to fight for and protect the interests of the unemployed and disadvantaged during this period, the unemployed themselves did not acquiesce silently to political attacks and cuts in relief payments. The justification for a campaign of mass extra-parliamentary activity during this period was evident, for as Miliband stated:

> Given the fact that Britain ... in 1931 [had] one of the richest ruling classes in the world, it is surely amazing that there were actually found rational men to argue that the saving of a few million pounds a year on the miserable pittances allowed to unemployed men and women and their children was the essential condition of British solvency.
>
> (Miliband 1972: 185)

Initially, in the early 1920s, the NUWM worked hard for Labour candidates, and it had high expectations when the first Labour government was elected in 1924. However, when the Labour Party showed no signs of fighting for working-class interests and defending the unemployed, there were calls for the development of an independent organization which would co-operate with the Labour movement, but would also refuse to subordinate its own interests to their leaders. In 1921 this led to the creation of the NUWM which was the first permanent organization set up specifically to defend the rights and standards of living of the unemployed by organizing and using collective action to protect working-class living standards. It was formed out of a London group led by three communists, Wal Hannington, Percy Haye and Jack Holt. However, it was Hannington who was the effective leader of the movement through the inter-war years. The oath of membership was: 'never to cease from active strife until capitalism is abolished', and by the time the NUWM was wound up in 1943, Hannington estimated that around 1 million people had passed through its ranks.

Although initially the NUWM was small and mainly London-based, as unemployment rose the organization grew, and its extra-parliamentary activities began to make the human problems of unemployment visible to the public in a way no parliamentary representation could. The aims of the organization can be summarized in six points. First, actively fighting unemployment by forcing the issue of unemployment and benefit cuts on to the national political stage. Second, emphasizing the links between the unemployed and those in work facing attacks on their wages and conditions. Third, posing demands on the state and the national polity, to 'expose' the inhumanity of capitalism, stressing that a system based on profit could not adequately meet the needs of the working class and that a new social system was necessary. Fourth, bringing pressure to bare on local PACs and forcing them to be more generous with their relief. Fifth, offering a legal and advisory network that would help workers threatened with benefit cuts or removal. And, finally, on occasion organizing a range of leisure and sporting activities. These aims were carried through in a myriad of ways, but the most enduring image was associated with its organization of national hunger marches.

The NUWM organized national hunger marches to London in 1922/3, 1929, 1932, 1934 and 1936. The marchers came from all over the country and represented a range of occupations. During the first hunger march in 1922 there were:

> Iron-and-steel workers from Scotland ... ship-yard workers of the Tyne, shipwrights of Barrow-in-Furness, dockers and seamen of Liverpool, iron-ore miners of Cumberland, cotton operatives of Lancashire, coal-miners of the South Wales valleys, engineers and mechanics from the Midlands, labourers from all parts of Britain.
> (Kingsford 1982: 33)

Each marcher was enrolled and swore an oath to: 'The general uplifting of the working class as a whole until emancipation from the clutches of a decaying system of society based upon Rent, Interest and Profit is achieved' (ibid.: 34).

The aim of the march was to raise the problem of unemployment and demand a meeting with the Prime Minister, Bonar Law, to demand work or maintenance at full trade union rates. The first marchers left Aberdeen in October and were soon joined on the road by contingents from across the country. They arrived in London on 15 November and prepared to march to the city centre and a massive reception from the workers and unemployed of the city. Bonar Law refused to meet representatives of the march, so the demonstrators stayed (some returning home and being replaced by substitutes) until 20 February 1923. The focus of the 1929 march was the iniquities of the Not Genuinely Seeking Work Test, while the 1932 march was in order to raise demands on the Labour Party to use their office to protect the poor. Among the NUWM's demands were:

Raise the benefit scales of the unemployed.

Remove the 'not genuinely seeking work' clause.

Restore to benefit all unemployed persons who were disqualified under the previous government's administration.

No disqualifications unless suitable employment at trade union rates has been offered and turned down.

A shorter working day, without loss of pay.

Adequate pensions for all workers over 60 years of age.

(Taken from Kingsford 1982: 114)

It is here that we most clearly see the politics of 'transitional demands' at work in the NUWM's activities.

During the marches, the unemployed were subject to strict discipline on the road and the movement was highly organized. For example, each contingent had a finance sub-committee and a treasurer to ensure that collections and donations were properly handled, and arrangements were made concerning food and accommodation. Nevertheless, marchers experienced hardship and had to make sacrifices in order to participate in hunger marches. These were related to poverty and the fact that the state bureaucracy often penalized marchers financially and attempted to make their lives as difficult as possible while they were 'on the road'. The marchers themselves needed a travelling card from their local labour exchange, but they first had to prove that they were marching in search of work. There were also concerns regarding the families of the unemployed who would be left to depend on the Board of Guardians, who might be hostile and refuse to provide outdoor relief. In such instances, funds had to be raised to support wives and children. On the road money for food was raised and meals and accommodation obtained where they could be found. Marchers experienced greatly differing responses from local communities and local authorities as they marched to London. In some instances they received a warm and generous welcome with adequate sleeping accommodation and nutritious meals. Some Boards of Guardians were sympathetic to their plight and offered them board and lodging. In some cases Boards of Guardians in poorer boroughs claimed they couldn't afford relief beyond the barest minimum, and some of these openly stated their opinion that maintenance should be paid for by the government, and supported the marchers by providing clothing and boots and paying for their lodgings in the workhouse. Other guardians treated them as vagrants; they subjected them to harsh and degrading treatment and only afforded the most pitiful provision in an attempt to get rid of the marchers by providing the bare legal minimum in terms of food and accommodation. Thus, some marchers were relatively well-clothed, fed and provided for while marching, whereas others lacked sufficient clothing and footwear and were ill-prepared for the rigours of marching in cold, wet and windy conditions, often contracting throat and chest ailments.

During the first hunger march the unemployed often received a warm and hospitable welcome from Trades Councils and Labour Councils who met the cost of food and accommodation in spite of hostility from the Ministry of Health. They also received support from the local unemployed. In contrast, the fourth hunger march, staged in March 1932, against the means test and a 10 per cent cut in benefits faced a much more co-ordinated, rigorous and harsh state response. The NUWM had made strenuous efforts to form reception committees along the routes and this proved successful. These committees, comprising of councillors, Co-op activists, Labour Party members, trade unionists, members of the Independent Labour Party, representatives of the churches and the Communist Party, offered support in the form of food, accommodation and entertainment, and organized a crowd of supporters if trouble with the police or the authorities was anticipated. But even so the marchers still experienced victimization, intimidation and violence from the police and the Poor Law authorities.

As well as the hunger marches, the NUWM also organized many local marches to PACs, to workhouses and to factories to hold factory-gate meetings. Local administration of benefits meant that these were a vital mechanism to bring pressure on local guardians. For example, in Birkenhead in September 1932 approximately 10,000 marched to the Birkenhead PAC to demand an increase in the scales of relief. During the march several people were arrested, and two days later another demonstration was held to demand the release of those arrested. Fighting broke out between demonstrators and police and the atmosphere intensified as the protests continued. On the fourth day the PAC made concessions, signalling a significant victory for the protesters.

The NUWM also led the movement against labour camps and was influential in refuting political arguments put forward to justify such developments, stressing that they were part of a wider strategy to create a large pool of cheap labour to undercut the position of the employed worker. It arranged meetings where letters of 'invitation' to attend labour camps were publicly burned. Similarly, the long-term unemployed faced difficulty in paying rent and bills, and another aspect to its campaign involved various measures to resist evictions (see McShane and Smith 1976; Damer, this volume). The stress on the 'unity' of the working class and a politics based on the development of 'socialism from below' meant activists of the NUWM were involved in many other local 'community', welfare and industrial campaigns including marches and demonstrations against the British Union of Fascists, who tried to actively recruit from among the unemployed.

The perceived threat to the state that the NUWM represented is emphasized by the hostility and repression which it faced. Its members were portrayed as criminals and communists, financed from Moscow. Police spies operated throughout the movement, bans were placed on demonstrations, and the police were given greater powers over the routing of marches. All marches faced close police scrutiny, and violence against marchers and demonstrators was a common occurrence, with civilian casualties across the country far outnumbering those of the police. In the four day confrontation in Birkenhead mentioned above, the police went around working-class neighbourhoods smashing windows and assaulting anyone they believed to be involved in the demonstrations. During this period the entire branch of the NUWM was arrested. In total forty-five protesters were eventually tried and two local NUWM leaders were sentenced to two years in prison. National leaders of the movement were also harassed, tried and sentenced for various offences. In March 1932 the bulk of the national leadership of the NUWM were imprisoned. Hannington was gaoled for three months for 'inciting the police'. These measures were intended to remove the most experienced leaders of the NUWM from the political scene, but while successful at this level, the disruptions did not stop the NUWM functioning – the involvement of large numbers of activists, across the country, provided a ready-made network of 'leaders' in a variety of localities.

The government also used administrative means to disrupt hunger marches and harass activists. For example, the Ministry of Labour told officials that they should refuse payment of unemployment benefit to marchers as they were not available to sign on for work, and the police were told to assist officials in enforcing these regulations. In this context it is perhaps worth mentioning that although the Jarrow march remains the best-known of all the marches against unemployment in the 1920s and 1930s, it was a relatively small affair which was organized by the town council to contrast with and set itself apart from the NUWM's marches and spirit of political militancy. It was a march sanctioned and supported by Labour Party and Trade Union leaders, various other politicians, and even Conservative MPs provided hospitality for the marchers as they made their way to London. The Jarrow Crusade was the respectable face of protest against the 'moral' problem of unemployment and hardship, organized and orchestrated by various official organizations; whereas the hunger marches were the demonstrations of the unemployed themselves, demanding the right to work and the right to benefits at a level to sustain more than mere existence.

The NUWM also offered help and advice to the unemployed over the level of benefits and relief eligibility, and represented them at tribunals. During the 1930s the NUWM's legal department began to function effectively, and it expanded enormously as unemployment increased and legislation became more complex. It had immense experience and expertise regarding National Insurance questions, and helped the unemployed to cope with the various relief bodies to ensure that benefit entitlement was met. This was an intimidating and complicated process as the unemployed had to defend themselves before courts of referees under the 'genuinely seeking work' clause which involved intense interrogation. Nevertheless, the NUWM did, at times, achieve results. For example, in some cases, cuts were restored, extra allowances won, and benefits were raised in line with neighbouring committees. Such detailed work with and on-behalf of the unemployed helps to explain the movement's strength: the daily struggles and battles were the necessary foundation on which the larger national campaigns could be built.

Finally, the NUWM also provided social activities for the unemployed and their families. For example, during the 1930s the NUWM leadership organized large-scale social events such as countryside rambles, children's parties and football matches – although the Communist Party criticized these events, claiming they encouraged 'passivity' and diverted the movement from mass agitation. But Hannington believed such activities were essential to build and maintain local relationships and maintain the spirit of activists in the movement.

The membership of the NUWM varied in terms of numbers and objectives during the 1920s and 1930s. It reached a peak in 1933, with high levels of activity taking place during this year. Although the average member only had a fleeting association with the movement in order to get better treatment from bureaucrats and improve benefits, for others, NUWM activity was a practical expression of a commitment to the wider struggle for socialism. The NUWM achieved many successes at both a local and a national level and they ensured that the unemployed in the crisis years could not be ignored or merely offered crumbs of sympathy. The organization activated thousands in the struggle against unemployment and the fight for a fairer society and it did so without adequate resources and in the face of opposition from, not just the state and the ruling class, but often the official layers of the labour and trade union movement. It is a fine example of people's ability to fight and struggle for a better world in the face of the most severe personal circumstances.

Conclusion

Our intention in this chapter has not been to 'measure' the Labour leaders of the 1920s and 1930s against some abstract revolutionary judgement. These leaders were not revolutionaries, they never claimed to be. Neither do we argue that Labour is not a party of reform; it clearly is – though whether it delivers reforms while in government is a separate matter. In 1945 a number of elements came together to produce a reforming Labour government, but in the 1920s and 1930s and indeed again at the end of the twentieth century, the Labour Party can be characterized as a reformist party unable to deliver significant reforms because their priority was (and is) to cure the economic problems of British capital in the name of the 'national interest'. The consequence is that the Labour Party pursued a strategy which pitted it against its own electoral constituency.

Our case is that, faced with the crisis of mass unemployment in the 1920s and 1930s, the labour movement was divided over the appropriate strategy to pursue. For the Labour Party leadership in government and in opposition, the goal was the economic recovery of British capitalism, and thus strategies to deal with unemployment were structured around re-establishing profitability. Thus, as we noted above, the approach became one of reducing government spending and attacking the unemployed. Of course, the suffering of the unemployed could still be portrayed as a national problem, but it was a 'moral' problem faced by a minority whose salvation would come when the economy returned to boom conditions. In these circumstances, hunger marches and other demonstrations were unnecessary and unwelcome. Politics was viewed by those in power as something which should be left to parliamentarians.

For the NUWM, unemployment was an inevitable consequence of capitalism, and, faced with its inexorable rise, it argued that it was necessary to redirect the vast wealth of British capital and the ruling class to maintain the living standards of the unemployed. The NUWM stressed the shared interests and concerns of those in work and those out of work and 'class' was emphasized as a unifying social and political concept, bringing together the oppressed and exploited. Calls for the redirection of resources were raised as a series of 'transitional demands' which would allow Communists, grass-roots Labour members and non-aligned activists to work together in the various unemployed struggles. The aim was to involve as many unemployed workers in a militant campaign for social reform and improvement and to stress the common class interest of the unemployed and employed worker.

The politics shaping the response of the Labour leadership and the NUWM can both be placed under the umbrella of 'socialism', but the contrasting goals, strategies and tactics of each reveal the 'two souls of socialism' in daily political practice. As a political goal, reform from above, administered by a few in the interests of the many, confines the majority in society to passivity and in this way reproduces the dominant relations of power and oppression. The politics of socialism from below is based on the possibility of working-class self-emancipation and so agitates for the widest involvement of the oppressed and exploited in the struggle for liberation. The two souls of socialism shape the terrain of debate and the strategic concerns of activists in the process of their social movement activity.

8 Housing and class struggles in post-war Glasgow

Charlie Johnstone

Introduction

In Chapter 5 in this volume, Seán Damer has highlighted the fact that class interests and class relations were crucial in structuring housing struggles on Clydeside in the early part of the twentieth century. The purpose of the following discussion is to extend this debate into a later period and emphasize the fact that the collective demands of the working class in Glasgow around the 'housing issue' remained a dominant feature of struggles by ordinary Glaswegians in the aftermath of the Second World War. To assess the importance of housing campaigns in the broader context of class struggle the focus of the discussion will concentrate on two early post-war housing campaigns. The first section will involve a brief description of working-class housing conditions in the early post-war period. This will be followed by a discussion of the emergence of the squatters' movement in the city around this time. The third section will provide an outline of a successful campaign to prevent the sale of an entire scheme (estate) of council housing in Glasgow in 1951–2. These are events that, despite their significance for the working class of Glasgow and beyond, have remained relatively 'hidden from history'. The concluding section will attempt to assess the significance of these struggles. It hardly needs to be said that, while the emphasis is on a particular 'locality', the debate will be located with reference to broader issues of housing policy within Britain which emerged during the period under discussion.

In one of a number of articles on housing in Glasgow the historian John Butt has claimed that action around housing during the post-war years amounted to a 'paler shade of Red Clydeside' (Butt 1978, 1987). Unfortunately, Butt never offers any definition of what he means by this and provides no detailed information to support such an assertion. In addition, his claim has rarely, if ever, been challenged despite the fact that anyone with a modicum of knowledge of working-class history would recognize this for the arrant nonsense that it is. Butt follows a long line of historians, alongside the parvenu class of 'housing experts', who regard the development of housing policy as part of a legislative and administrative process somehow separate from broader social and economic struggles which inevitably take place within class divided societies. Such analyses also ignore the significance of the demands and campaigns of working people to shape and influence social policy. The principal task here is to 'rescue' such struggles and make knowledge of their character available to a wider audience and place them in the wider context of class struggle.

Post-war housing conditions in Glasgow

It is now widely accepted that Glasgow has been beset with a working-class housing 'problem' since at least the mid-nineteenth century (see, for instance, Damer 1990; Gibb 1983; Pacione 1995). Indeed, it is a problem which still persists in the late 1990s, with the present City Council (in 1999) proposing to transfer the remaining local authority stock (around 160,000 dwellings) to private 'housing companies'. However, while each of these issues is generally known, it may come as some surprise to many with an interest in housing history and housing policy to learn the extent of the 'housing problem' in early post-war Glasgow.

It is important to acknowledge that, unlike many other British cities, or even the nearby town of Clydebank, Glasgow suffered very little in the way of bomb damage between 1939 and 1945. Nevertheless, the housing situation for the working class in Glasgow during this period was quite desperate, as evidenced by the assessment of the local Medical Officer of Health: 'It is estimated that some 100,000 houses will require to be built to replace unfit houses, to relieve overcrowding, and for general needs' (Glasgow Corporation 1943: 143). Indeed, some neighbourhoods still had an average of 700 persons per acre in 1951 (Damer 1990: 187). With the population of the city in 1951 standing at 1,090,000 there were around 100,000 people living in sub-let rooms, and 134,435 dwellings were judged to be overcrowded (44.2 per cent of the city's housing stock). Quite simply, in comparison with other British cities, the housing situation in Glasgow was abysmal, a fact recorded in the 1951 Census (see Table 8.1).

Table 8.1   Principal cities of Britain, statistics relating to housing conditions in 1951

City	% of dwellings with one or two rooms	% of population living at more than two persons per room	% of households lacking a fixed bath
Glasgow	41.5	24.4	50.1
Manchester	0.5	2.1	33.0
Birmingham	0.5	3.3	38.0
Leeds	2.0	2.6	28.0
Liverpool	1.1	6.0	36.0
London	2.7	2.5	44.0
Sheffield	0.6	2.5	45.0

Source: Census, 1951

The scale of the 'housing problem' in Glasgow during the post-war period led to conflict between the local and national state over ways to remedy the situation. Essentially, the dispute revolved around the issue of whether housing could be provided within the existing city boundaries or, alternatively, that large numbers of the population would have to be rehoused in new towns and housing schemes on the periphery of the city. The final outcome was a classic compromise which incorporated aspects of both plans, with the new towns of Cumbernauld and East Kilbride providing housing for Glasgow's skilled 'overspill' population and the four main peripheral housing schemes (Castlemilk, Drumchapel, Easterhouse and Pollok) generally accommodating the unskilled and semi-skilled sections of the local working class. The story of these events is now well recorded in the literature on the city (see, for instance, Gibb 1983; Worsdall 1979), but certain important working-class struggles around the housing issue during this period remain relatively unknown and it is to these events we now turn.

Property is for people: squatting in Glasgow

> Anything which threatens people's homes or their ability to obtain a home can immediately land a government in a great deal of trouble.
>
> (Blakemore 1998: 143)

In early post-war Britain the government did find itself in a 'great deal of trouble' over the housing issue, partly as a result of war-time restrictions on building. This took the form of thousands of properties being taken over by squatters, organized in the main by working-class and socialist organizations, with the additional support in some localities of prominent anarchists (Anning *et al.* 1980). The problem faced by many people after the Second World War was quite simply to do with homelessness and overcrowded living conditions. The circumstances surrounding the development of the squatters' movement in Glasgow (and elsewhere) are obviously connected to debates about the national housing problem and changes at the level of state power, with the emergence of the Keynesian welfare state; a fact clearly recognized by at least one Conservative politician during the war who made the following observation: 'if you do not give the people social reform, they are going to give you social revolution' (Hogg 1944). The aspirations of many working-class people for improvement in their standard of living helped to fuel the anger regarding the housing situation that many faced (see, for instance, Calder 1969). However, while acknowledging these important issues, the main purpose of this section is to describe the specific local factors pertaining to Glasgow in order to highlight the role of grass-roots activity and action around the provision of housing in the city.

For the working class of Glasgow, regardless of the promises of the post-war Labour government, housing in the city was, to say the least, scarce and overcrowded. In common with many other working-class towns and cities throughout Britain the working class of Glasgow took drastic action to alleviate their housing situation by occupying empty premises and organizing themselves into Defence Committees in a concerted effort to provide shelter for the homeless and those living in overcrowded accommodation. This activity was of an extra-parliamentary nature and was planned and organized from within the working class. As we will see, this type of action was also met with attempts by the state to assert political control of the events surrounding squatting.

Beginning in 1946, large numbers of working-class families began taking over various unoccupied properties throughout Glasgow, including churches, hotels, mansion houses, former warder's quarters at Barlinnie Prison, the Glasgow Press Club and a hospital. The squatters were supported by numerous working-class organizations, including tenants' associations, the remaining elements in the Independent Labour Party (ILP) and the local Communist Party. The working-class theatre group, Glasgow Unity Theatre, produced a seminal play (*The Gorbals Story*) which highlighted the plight of the homeless and was explicitly aimed at supporting the growing squatters' movement. The reasoning behind this support and the actual squatting itself was summed up very simply by one of those involved at the time:

> We are all decent working folk and we are desperate for some place in which to live. I have five children, their ages ranging from four to sixteen, and one of them being bedridden. During my married life I have only once had a sub-let house. My name has been on the Corporation waiting list for 11 years.
>
> (*Glasgow Herald*, 28 August 1946)

In other words, to gain one of the most basic of human needs, a shelter, working-class families had to take direct action and occupy buildings that were often without heating, lighting or sanitary conveniences. There was no council housing available for them, and had not been for some years. The squatters and their families moved into vacant properties and chalked their names on the doors of tenement apartments that had been lying disused for up to ten years (this became a common way of 'booking-in'). On one occasion a prominent member of the Communist Party worked overnight with a mash hammer and stone chisel and cut a way through the back wall of a vacant property to allow families to enter undetected. While contemporary moralistic discourses within social policy would label such individuals as part of the so-called 'underclass', in 1946 such people managed to attain partial support from some unusual quarters, as the following suggests:

> In a country so law-abiding as Great Britain it is always refreshing when the people take the law into their own hands on an issue on which the spirit of justice, if not its letter, is so eminently on their side.
>
> (*The Economist*, 24 August 1946)

By the autumn of 1946 squatting had become firmly established as a central part of the working-class struggle for decent affordable housing within Glasgow. The aspirations of working people for a better future and decent housing were being tested through the inadequacies which prevailed during the early years of the welfare state. In such a situation, many working-class people took the only action available to them to alleviate their situation and by August 1946 the number of squatters in Glasgow had increased to around 1,500 families.

The actions of the squatters were met with a predictable response from property owners, the Corporation of Glasgow and central government. In late August and early September 1946 a number of squatters and their families were forcefully evicted from properties throughout the city. In September a special meeting of the Glasgow Property Owners and Factors Association expressed concern at the government's lack of action in protecting private property:

> The government, said a spokesman, ... have found an apparent solution so far as their own property is concerned, but they have signally failed to do anything about the invasion of private property by squatters.
>
> (*Glasgow Herald*, 6 September 1946)

The 'solution' referred to in the above quotation was the government's decision to allow squatters throughout Britain to occupy Nissen huts on former military camps. Many people had been occupying these camps for months, running them on a non-profit-making basis until new local authority housing became available. The government's proposal was to convert such camps into 'temporary' housing, though many people lived in such camps until the late 1950s. However, aware of the contradictory nature of such a policy option, the Joint Under-Secretary of State for Scotland, George Buchanan, withdrew the proposal, and argued that squatters would neither be allowed to run their own camps or co-operate with the government or local authorities in running them. Buchanan also used this opportunity to make a forthright condemnation of squatting in general saying that 'such invasions of private premises are a challenge to the law of the land. In the interests of the vast majority of law-abiding citizens the law must take its course'.

The law was already taking its course in Glasgow. In mid-September 1946 the first arrests of squatters were made in the city during a number of early morning raids.[1] The squatters were charged with trespassing, a criminal offence in Scotland since the period of the Highland Clearances. The local state also resorted to disconnecting gas and electricity supplies to premises in order to force the squatters out. It has to be remembered that these actions were taken under the auspices of the first majority Labour government, and that the interests of 'private' property were seen to be more important than those of working-class people. While the squatters had directed their attention to 'public' premises, such as the former Army camps, they represented a lesser threat to the law and to the principle of private property. Once the squatters began to take over privately-owned property the state, and its agents, used all of the power at their disposal to support those landlords whose interests were threatened. Aneurin Bevan, the minister responsible for housing at the time, summed up these views simply when he stated that while 'he sympathised with the squatters he could not allow them to take command' (quoted in Foot 1975: 81).

By October 1946 there were around 7,000 people occupying former Army camps in Scotland and another 46,335 in England and Wales. However, the government was not solely concerned with the activities of squatters, more important in this context, and why Bevan probably did not want them to 'take command', was the involvement of Communist Party members in the movement.

The Communist Party (CP) was actively involved in helping squatters to take over private property, in the first instance on a small scale in Glasgow, but more particularly in London. The activity of the CP in London reached its zenith with the highly publicized, and perhaps opportunistic, ploy of advertising the availability of unfurnished flats in newspapers. The flats in question were actually empty 'luxury flats' at Duchess of Bedford House in Kensington, and were owned by a number of peers. The CP managed to bring together a number of squatters and their families and move them into these flats in what became known as the 'great Sunday squat'. The squatters immediately elected an emergency committee to represent themselves in negotiations with the local council. A number of Cabinet meetings were held to discuss the matter which led to claims of impending 'anarchy', an obvious indication that the government recognized the potential political threat of such activity. The leaders of the CP were also clearly aware of the political potential of this type of social protest, and expressed their critique of the state's dilemma in unambiguously class terms:

> All this talk about the liberty of the individual and the sacred rights of private property, and about the forces of anarchy that have been let loose is merely a cover for panic attempts to preserve the system of rich and poor, of homeless and those with more than one home. These seizures will stop when local authorities carry out their responsibilities to the homeless, and when the Government overrides those Tory-dominated local councils.
>
> (Harry Pollitt, General Secretary of the Communist Party, quoted in Mahon 1978: 320)

In any event, the state acted swiftly to curtail these developments. Five members of the CP involved in this particular campaign were arrested on serious charges of 'criminal conspiracy' and conspiring to incite trespass, a clear indication that the Labour government would not tolerate the expropriation of private property. Following eviction orders served by the High Court, the squatters eventually vacated the premises, but were also found guilty of trespass and 'bound over' for two years.

Alongside this type of legal repression and coercion of the squatting movement there were a number of 'short-term' policy responses, as Short has noted:

> Dwellings were requisitioned, premises converted, repairs hurriedly made to houses and prefabricated dwellings were constructed. By 1948 almost 125,000 'prefabs' had been built. Although built as a short-term solution, many of them lasted into the 1970s.
>
> (Short 1982: 42)

However, the squatting movement provided a necessary stimulant to the many dilatory local authorities and did not end at this point; many people in Glasgow continued to occupy Army camps and condemned properties throughout the 1940s and, in some cases, through to the late 1950s. Indeed the local state was still trying to evict families of squatters from condemned properties as late as 1959. In one case the demolition squad refused to carry out their work until the families agreed to move out. It must also be remembered that the squatters' own experience of their living conditions was not always a happy one, as one contemporary account suggests:

> Life is a fight, not only against authority, dirt, cold, damp, heat, illness and rats, but against one's own apathy. Families begin to crack at different periods. On the faces of some there is a look of strain, of controlled despair, such as soldiers show when they have seen too much action. At the camp committees they say, quite plainly, there is a limit to human endurance. They live near the edge of that limit, fearing that some day they will slip over.
>
> (*New Statesman and Nation*, 1 March 1952)

Despite such an appalling set of circumstances these people did not 'slip over', and along with tenants' associations and other labour organizations in Glasgow they expanded their protests against the cuts in the building programme which resulted from the reduced financial allocation given to the city in the government's 1947 Housing Programme.

By highlighting the nature and extent of the 'housing problem' in Glasgow and elsewhere, the squatters appealed to the aspirations of a radicalized working-class population in post-war Britain. They continued to put pressure on the state to fulfill the promises which it had made or, in the case of housing, it had not made in 1945 (the Labour government had reneged on the commitment to set up a Ministry of Housing contained in their 1945 election manifesto). The simple lesson from this case is that the provision of adequate, affordable rented accommodation for the working class was not an inevitable development of the post-war welfare state. Like earlier struggles over housing issues, the provision of decent housing for the working classes in the post-war years was one that had to be fought hard for and would not have been successful without the involvement of thousands of working-class people 'on the ground' taking direct action in a struggle for a basic human need.

Whose houses are these?: The Merrylee Road campaign

In its 1945 election manifesto, the Conservative Party became the first British political organization to explicitly put forward the idea of a 'property owning democracy' and to emphasize the 'superiority' of owner occupation over other forms of housing tenure. Throughout the period of the 1945–51 Labour government the slogan of a 'property owning democracy' came to symbolize the Conservative opposition's alternative housing policies. This approach became more apparent when the Conservatives were elected in 1951 with Harold MacMillan (Minister for Housing) clearly stating his government's goal: 'We wish to see the widest possible distribution of property. We think that, of all forms of property suitable for such distribution house property is one of the best' (Harold MacMillan, quoted in *Hansard* 1951, vol. 494: 2227–354).

The Conservative government issued a general consent which enabled local authorities to carry out house sales. The idea of a 'property owning democracy' was to become a political reality, or so it was assumed. With hindsight this was the beginning of a political and ideological battle over the nature of state-provided housing which was to last for around thirty years and culminated in the 1980 ('the right to buy') Housing Act. However, it is important to point out that the reality of Conservative housing policy in the 1950s was actually somewhat different, as more local authority houses were built under the Conservatives than under the 1945–51 Labour government.

While MacMillan was announcing his 'housing crusade' such a policy was actually being pursued with vigour by the so-called Progressive (i.e. Tory) controlled Corporation of Glasgow. In May 1951, the Housing Committee of Glasgow Corporation first discussed a government allocation of 500 houses to be built under building licences for sale to approved categories of purchasers. One vital criterion introduced here was the ability to pay a down payment of £250 and rental of around £3 per week. Despite the fact that there were over 100,000 people on the housing waiting list, the Progressive council was clearly intent on giving priority to building houses for sale rather than to let and limiting access to those who could afford to pay. The purpose of this approach to the provision of housing became apparent on 5 September 1951, when the leader of the council put forward the proposal to offer for sale a whole housing scheme which had originally been built to rent. This was the first time that any local authority in Britain had attempted to do such a thing. The events surrounding the proposal to sell the houses at the Merrylee Road scheme were summed up briefly in one contemporary account:

> The Progressives proposed to offer a number of Council-built houses for sale. This was a move of ordinary justice and ordinary common sense. ... In vain did Progressive candidates argue that every house sold was a relief to the rates, and in vain did they point out that a remarkable number of Socialist Councillors were enjoying rent subsidy. There were demonstrations and threats of strikes, and the Socialists were returned on the claim that it was the blackest reaction to interfere with the sacred principle of some-thing for nothing. It was a curious and saddening instance of how far bitterness and bigotry have penetrated the proletarian mind.
>
> (Brogan 1952: 216)

This account, by a contemporary right-wing commentator, is not only derisory and malicious but, as will become clear, totally inaccurate. Indeed, there were strikes to support the campaign and people did not want 'something for nothing', what they wanted was council houses they could rent rather than housing for sale.

The Progressives in Glasgow were merely acting out the stated aims of the Conservative Party at both local and national level. Their plans to sell the houses at Merrylee Road, on the south-side of Glasgow, were initially couched in economic terms. Their attack on the financing of council housing was part of a wider debate on housing policy, for instance, a leading article in the *London Times*, commenting on housing subsidies, suggested that the new procedure will 'save public funds even if it does not increase the volume of new housing' (*London Times*, 29 November 1951). However, for the Progressives in Glasgow, there were additional ideological motives behind the proposed sale of the Merrylee Road houses, as evidenced in a City Assessor's report:

> the houses were superior in construction and finish to houses being built and sold by private builders and were situated in what from a 'valuation' viewpoint was the best residential district in the city. The cost of upkeep should be low and the amenity value high for many years. If all the houses were sold to private owners they should retain also the value appertaining to a 'good address'.
>
> (Quoted in *Glasgow Herald*, 29 November 1951)

What was being asserted was that the houses at Merrylee Road were not only of a very high quality but had potential for future accumulation purposes for Tory supporters. The dominant view that was constructed by the Progressives, therefore, was that 'superior' houses at a 'good address' were not to be made available to working-class tenants for rent. This 'residential district' was to be ordered in such a way as to restrict entry to those 'respectable' enough to buy such houses at prices equivalent to properties in the private market. In this respect the Progressives were attempting to bring about a fundamental change in the nature of housing provision by local authorities. In short, their belief was that good quality housing should not be subsidized, and for that they were described as 'the most reactionary local authority in Britain' (*Forward*, 8 December 1951). Protests were also forthcoming from private builders who, no doubt, feared the competition which could result from such a change in housing policy:

> The Corporation's idea to sell the houses to people with the money to buy them and so take the burden off the ratepayer is an admirable one, but if we got the licences we could do exactly the same thing.
>
> (John Lawrence,
> quoted in the *Bulletin and Scots Pictorial*, 7 September 1951)

However, this type of protest was mild in comparison with what was to follow. The first signs of unrest came from building workers when the Housing Convener sent a personal message of thanks to them in their pay packets for their productivity levels. The building workers on the large Cranhill site in the east end of the city were not impressed and responded accordingly:

> We think this is downright cheek and hypocrisy, viewing the recent decision pushed through by you to sell the 622 Merrylee houses which are being built by our fellow-workers and were originally intended for rent.
>
> (Ned Donaldson, building workers' shop steward,
> quoted in *Glasgow Herald*, 4 December 1951)

The challenge to the proposal to sell the Merrylee houses was beginning. On 3 December 1951 a meeting called by the joint-shop stewards committee at Weir's Engineering, a firm situated near to the Merrylee site, decided to organize a demonstration in George Square on 6 December, the day that the full Corporation were to debate the proposal to sell off the Merrylee houses. The meeting brought together over 100 delegates from twenty organizations, mostly building and engineering trade unionists, representatives from tenants' associations, women's groups and Labour Party branches and three Labour councillors. The organizers of this meeting also proposed that a delegation of workers should seek to put forward their views in opposition to the proposed sale of the Merrylee houses to the Housing Committee.

This gives an indication of the fact that the proposed sale of the Merrylee Road houses was regarded as a major challenge to the labour movement's advocacy of state provided housing for rent. What also emerges in this context is the conflict between those who believed that change could come through debating within the council chamber and those who advocated direct and grass-roots action from the base of the working class. These opposing strategies continued throughout the campaign in a manner consistent with alternative approaches to agitation evident within working-class organizations on similar campaigns, then and now.

On the day of the full council meeting around 5,000 people took part in the demonstration against the sale of the Merrylee Road houses. Building workers across the city had decided to go on strike for the day to support the demonstration. They were supported by workers from the shipyards, transport workers, railway workers,

engineers from Weirs and from Mavor and Coulson's heavy engineering works in Bridgeton in the east end of Glasgow which had been
closed down for the day. Alongside these trade unionists were a large
number of representatives from tenants' associations and women's
groups across the city.

Some of the demonstrators at the front of the march tried to storm
the City Chambers but were prevented from doing so by a heavy
police presence. However, a number of the demonstrators managed to
gain access and delayed the start of the meeting, and a deputation
from Glasgow Trades' Council put forward the case against the sale of
the houses at Merrylee Road. Despite the numerous protests from
workers' organizations, the Progressive controlled Corporation voted
in favour of the sale going ahead.

Shortly after this decision, working-class organizations began
daubing the streets with chalk and paint to advertise public meetings
across the city. It was around this time that a Joint Committee to stop
the sale of the Merrylee Road houses was formed, under the auspices
of engineering workers at Weirs. However, divisions emerged between
those who favoured campaigns of direct action, and traditionalists in
the Labour Party who wanted to pursue the campaign through
debates in the City Chambers. This division became obvious at a rally
organized by the Labour Party on 12 December 1951. There were
around 2,000 people at the rally in St Andrew's hall, but the Labour
MPs present refused to support a proposal for more demonstrations
and strikes. The Labour Group on the Corporation also expressed
their opposition to such action, with one member declaring that 'the
Labour Group do not countenance any unofficial and unconstitu-
tional action on the industrial side' (Andrew Hood, Leader of the
Labour Group, quoted in the *Bulletin*, 14 December 1951).

The demonstration went ahead in any case with around 1,500
people taking part. Again, the deputations of workers were ignored
and the elected representatives had decided that the debate on the sale
of these council houses was to be conducted within the confines of
representative democracy. The Labour Group on the council were
obviously intent on retaining hegemonic control of the campaign and
favoured petitions and representations to the Corporation and the
Secretary of State for Scotland. An almost identical approach was
adopted by the Scottish Trade Union Congress (STUC). The
campaign against the sale continued along the same lines through late
1951 and the early months of 1952, as Donaldson and Forster suggest:

During the rest of December the campaign against the sale moved from the industrial area into the districts. Meetings in all the main areas were organised by tenants' associations, Labour Parties and Communist Parties. Large meetings were held in local halls, addressed by speakers from the Merrylee campaign committee. ... There was even an open-air bonfire meeting in the Partick area.

(Donaldson and Forster 1993: 21)

However, the proposed sale of these houses became a national issue when separate delegations from the STUC and Glasgow Labour MPs met with the Secretary of State for Scotland. The issue of the sale was also regarded by working-class organizations across Scotland as a threat to the whole notion of state provided housing for the working class and, if implemented in Glasgow, would eventually spread to other local authorities. In Glasgow another protest demonstration was organized for 30 January 1952. Despite the fact that Glasgow magistrates invoked the Public Order Act 1936 to ban the demonstration, around 2,000 marched to the City Chambers. Again their protests were ignored and the Progressives approved conditions set down by the Secretary of State for Scotland, who had now given his consent for the sale of the Merrylee houses to go ahead. At this stage the Progressives increased their attack on the concept of state provided housing, with council leader Alexander MacPherson Rait at the forefront:

in Glasgow 25 per cent of the houses available to let were municipal houses and 75 per cent were privately owned. The municipal houses carried a government subsidy, but since 1945 that had not met the gap between rent plus subsidy and the total cost. Between May 1946 and May 1951, £2,628,000 had been paid from the rates. That meant that 75 per cent of the people – those living in factor's houses – were subsidising those who had corporation houses.

(Quoted in the *Glasgow Herald*, 22 February 1952)

The ideology of the 'oversubsidized' council tenant was now being used with a vengeance to justify the sale of the houses. By the end of April 1952, eight of the houses at Merrylee Road had been processed for sale and a further ninety-six applications for purchase were being processed by the Corporation. However, the municipal elections were due to take place on 7 May and the Merrylee Road issue dominated the campaign. Working-class activists agitated throughout the election campaign, daubing the streets with slogans and campaigning outside polling booths on the day of the election. As a result, Labour gained power in Glasgow taking ten seats from the Progressives, to give them a majority of fifteen. The newly elected Labour leader's first statement was on the Merrylee issue when he indicated that the proposal to sell the houses would be reversed: 'We will take the earliest opportunity of making all the Merrylee houses which have not been sold available to those in want' (Andrew Hood, quoted in the *Bulletin*, 7 May 1952).

The Labour controlled Corporation had no alternative other than to reverse the decision. Those involved in direct action against the proposal had made sure that the Merrylee issue dominated the whole election campaign, and it was on the basis of making these houses available for letting that Labour were elected. Working-class agitation had brought the issue of housing provision to the fore and played a vital role in providing a challenge to the Progressive's proposals to sell the Merrylee houses.

The plan to sell the houses at Merrylee Road was reversed at a full meeting of the Corporation on 29 May 1952. For the working-class and socialist organizations who had mobilized thousands of Glaswegians and held hundreds of meetings over some months this was a major achievement. It had enormous implications for housing policy, both in Glasgow and elsewhere; and it would be another thirty years before a serious proposal to sell-off council housing would be heard again.

Conclusion

It needs to be stated that the events referred to in the preceding discussion took place initially under the first majority Labour government and at a time when the welfare state was in its infancy. However, during this period class interests and class relations remained central to struggles over the provision of local authority housing to let. The provision of council housing, in Glasgow at least, did not represent an 'inevitable' and progressive step in policy-making.

The collective demands of the working class have been more decisive in the development of housing policy than has been acknowledged to date. While there may not have been a 'revolutionary moment' in Glasgow in the 1940s and 1950s, the campaign and struggle over housing conditions and housing provision remained at the top of the working-class political agenda, and it was a struggle which was quite clearly successful.

The reason that the events portrayed in this chapter were not 'insignificant' or only of interest to the people involved is that they were not interpreted by those working-class individuals and organizations who campaigned around squatting or the Merrylee Road issue as 'consumption' struggles. Instead they interpreted these events as part of the working-class struggle for the amelioration of working-class living conditions. It was a struggle which made links between workplace organizations and working-class 'communities' in a united campaign for decent, affordable, rented accommodation. They may not have been involved in a struggle with an identifiable 'class enemy', but throughout their campaigns they emphasized the fact that the state had a central role in providing housing for the working class. By taking forms of direct action to provide a shelter for their families, the squatters were challenging the rules relating to the use of 'private property'. It was only by taking such direct action that the state was eventually forced to allow people to occupy the Army camps. Both the squatting movement and the Merrylee campaign were led by 'organic intellectuals' of the working class, members of the Labour Party, the CP, tenants' representatives, women's groups and trade unionists. They drew upon a rich associational life of diverse organizations, informed by socialist perspectives, to fight for the social improvement of working-class living conditions. To their credit, the people involved in both of the campaigns outlined in this chapter, made a major contribution to class struggle around housing issues in the post-war years.

As the New Labour government in the late 1990s continues the previous Conservative government's housing policy of privatization and transfer from council control to the private rented sector, the housing campaigns of the post-war years provide some important lessons for those trying to resist such processes and maintain a council housing sector committed to housing for need not profit.

Note

1   This was a tactic first used by Glasgow's private landlords to control overcrowding of 'ticketed houses' in the nineteenth century. Basically, this was a process whereby the local sanitary police would raid houses in the middle of the night to check that the officially stipulated number of occupants resided in the premises. If the numbers exceeded the law then tenants would be taken to court, fined and often evicted.

9 The struggle for abortion rights

Sue Clegg and Rita Gough

Introduction

Abortion has been used over the centuries as one way for women to control their fertility, and in the twentieth century struggles over abortion rights have had an immense significance on women's lives and on social welfare. The question is not whether women have abortions, but the conditions under which they do so. It is these conditions which signal that abortion is a class issue. Class differentials in access to safe abortion can be seen most clearly prior to the legalization of abortion in Britain and the United States. For the minority of rich women who could afford the services of physicians, in either semi-legal or illegal circumstances, abortion was medically safe and the risks of prosecution were slim. However, for the vast majority of women, both in Britain and in the States, the legal status of abortion meant unsafe, self-inflicted abortions or intervention by non-medical practitioners, whose competency varied, as well as the threat of legal prosecution or humiliation by the authorities. The rallying cry 'We remember' resonates with the experiences of these women and encompasses high mortality rates, the misery of botched abortions, and bearing unwanted children in often desperate economic circumstances (Ross 1998).

It is often assumed that abortion, and the struggle for abortion rights, was and is primarily a feminist issue. However, we will argue that an analysis of the history suggests a more complex story. Our analysis highlights some of the limitations of feminist theory and politics, as well as emphasizing the central importance of women's oppression in terms of understanding society. The importance of committed scholarship has long been recognized by feminists and socialists, and has now gained acceptance in the broader academic community as the biases of previously assumed objective scholarship have been exposed. Analysis of the conditions of struggle and their outcomes informs practice, and we write as committed socialists who have been active in the struggles described. This chapter should therefore be read as an intervention in the debates about abortion rights as well as an analysis of events.

Our approach is both historical and comparative, and we locate abortion struggles within an analysis of broader socio-economic and political trends. The comparative dimension is crucial. Some underlying structural conditions affecting the lives of women are the same, most notably the secular trend towards increased women's participation in the workforce, increased access to all levels of education, and a general extension of civil and political rights to women. These broader trends account for the overall resilience of popular support for legal abortion and opposition to recriminalization, despite ideological attacks from the right.

There are, however, significant differences in abortion politics between Britain and the United States. The different political systems of these two countries determined the legislative framework for legalization of abortion. More important, the differences in political culture have profoundly affected the type and scale of mobilization in favour of abortion. In Britain the Abortion Act 1967 was initially passed as a piece of liberalizing, lobby group, legislation. However, the defence of the 1967 Act from attack involved trade unionists, socialists and Labour Party activists, as well as women influenced by the women's movement. In the United States the 1973 Supreme Court judgment which legalized abortion was influenced by feminist activity through the courts. However, the subsequent ferocity of the ideological assault on abortion rights in the United States has not been paralleled in Britain. Moreover, the weaknesses of the movement in defence of abortion in the States is in part a consequence of the failure of the women's movement, especially the National Organization for Women (NOW), to connect with women and men outside its largely middle-class, white constituency (Solinger 1998). Our analysis, therefore, carries within it implications for practice, as well an understanding of the events described.

The chapter is structured to allow for both the historical and comparative dimensions. The first section looks at the social and economic conditions in the first half of the twentieth century in Britain and demonstrates the unequal access for women to safe, legal abortion. The second section looks at the campaigns which resulted in the 1967 Abortion Act. The third section deals with attacks on the Act and the mobilizations in its defence, concentrating particularly on the campaign against the introduction of a bill by John Corrie in 1979 and David Alton's 1988 Abortion Amendment Bill. The comparison between the two campaigns mounted in defence of the Abortion Act shows the way in which the general political climate affects the level of mobilization. The fourth section takes a comparative perspective with regard to the situation in the United States. Finally, in the conclusion, we return to the theoretical themes set out in this introduction.

Abortion in the first half of the twentieth century in Britain

From 1861 abortion in Britain was a misdemeanour and anyone procuring an abortion, including the woman, could be sentenced to life imprisonment. There was no provision for medical abortion. In 1929 the Infant Life Preservation Act made abortion unlawful except where it could be proved to have been done to preserve the life of the mother. An exemplary prosecution in 1938 of a doctor involved in the medical abortion on a 14-year-old multiple rape victim, established a liberal interpretation of the 1929 Act which protected doctors (and their mainly rich clients) from prosecution. From 1929 an affluent minority of women had access to safe, if semi-legal, medical abortion through private practitioners. For most women, however, attempts to terminate an unwanted pregnancy were dangerous. The majority of abortions were illegal under the 1929 Act, and were obtained through backstreet abortionists or through horrific attempts to self-induce.

The organized political struggle for legal abortion dates from 1936 with the formation of the Abortion Law Reform Association (ALRA) by Janet Chance, Stella Browne and Alice Jenkins. Most of the original committee members were also in the Labour Party, and were active in the birth control and suffrage movements. Browne had been an influential member of the British Communist Party (BCP) until 1923 when she resigned because the Party refused to follow post-revolutionary Russia's 1920 policy of legalizing abortion on demand. This was the first country to legalize abortion and allow abortion on request. The BCP's position, in contrast to Browne's, reflected an inability to distinguish between Malthusian population policies and women's demands for self-determination of their fertility (Rowbotham 1977). Chance, Browne and Jenkins also identified themselves as 'new feminists', supporting sexual fulfilment of women and men, in contrast to pre-suffrage feminists who tended to advocate male sexual abstinence. Female sexual reformers recognized that voluntary motherhood should be a choice for all women, to release them from the unnecessary tyranny of unwanted pregnancies. For the founding members of ALRA, political and social reforms were inseparable from sexual reform, allowing women to decide if and when to have children.

Fertility rates had started to decline as early as the 1870s and there is evidence that abortion was common practice (Pugh 1992). By the 1930s there was political concern over a continuing decline in fertility rates especially in middle-class women. However, fertility varied not only between classes but also within the working class where there was a correlation between levels of fertility and female employment. In Lancashire where textile mills relied on female labour, fertility was markedly lower than in mining districts with low levels of female employment (Pugh 1992). In contrast to improving infant mortality, maternal mortality increased from 4.83 per 1,000 births in 1923 to 5.94 in 1933 (Pugh 1992). The generally accepted explanation for this increase is malnutrition due to the appalling conditions of working-class life exacerbated by the inter-war depression (Davin 1978). However, deaths attributable to infections following abortion also exacted a considerable toll (Graves 1994). Nor was childbearing much safer, as Dora Russell and Frida Laski on a speaking tour in Durham were appalled to discover: 'It was four times as dangerous to bear a child as to work in a coal-mine, and mining was held to be men's most dangerous trade' (quoted in Simms 1992).

Working-class women relied on abortions, either self-induced or assisted. All manner of dangerous and inappropriate instruments, such as meat skewers, douches and concoctions, including iodine and lethal poisons, were easily purchased from chemists, tobacconists and herbalist shops. Alternatively, they answered advertisements for 'remedies', sought the services of quacks or found a sympathetic female known to assist with abortions. Despite the obvious dangers, abortion was a common and necessary means of birth control which working-class women considered neither criminal nor morally wrong (McLaren 1978; Graves 1994). It was the birth control movement which drew a distinction between pre- and post-conception methods which was not shared by working-class women, or indeed observed by commercial suppliers who profited from such sales (Brookes 1988). Other means of birth control were largely inaccessible for working-class women who had little contact with the medical profession or birth control clinics. Clinics only provided contraception to married women who suffered poor health and therefore their services were not generally available (Pugh 1992).

In contrast, it was easier for middle-class women to safely end an unwanted pregnancy. The Infant Life Preservation Act 1929, which allowed abortion if a woman's life was in danger, and the Bourne judgment in 1938, which ruled that no clear distinction could be drawn between threat to life and threat to health, allowed a legal loophole for widening the terms of abortion. However, this loophole could only be exploited by women with the means to afford to pay a private medical practitioner to perform a discrete and safe termination.

The growing concern over maternal mortality and illegal abortions was the driving force behind the government setting up a number of inquiries, including the Birkett committee in 1937. From the evidence presented the committee estimated that around 60,000 backstreet abortions took place annually, resulting in around 500 deaths each year (Simms 1992). The committee considered the reasons for abortions as primarily influenced by economic factors, finding that working-class women were often the primary wage earner in the face of large-scale male unemployment and grinding poverty. In these conditions it was not only desirable but necessary to restrict numbers of children. ALRA, in giving evidence to the committee, appealed for abortion reform on the basis of hardship cases, only Stella Browne argued for abortion on demand for all women in all cases 'without insolent inquisitions nor ruinous financial charges, nor tangles of red tape' (Rowbotham 1977: 159). She went on to point out that abortion was a safe procedure under the right conditions, and admitted speaking from her own experience (Russell 1977).

The activities of the ALRA were temporarily halted by the outbreak of the Second World War. Following the war, a number of key changes took place which gradually refuelled the struggle for legalized abortion. The most important of these changes was the establishment of the welfare state, for the first time ensuring the provision of free health care, education and the promise of full male employment. However, birth control methods, although more respectable, remained limited as they were not included in the National Health Service Act,[1] and deaths from illegal abortions continued. Unequal access to abortion remained as the new National Health Service (NHS) was much stricter in its application of the law than individual private physicians. Prior to the 1967 Act, only 5,700 abortions were carried out by the NHS compared to 15,000 privately (Francome 1986). As a consequence, as late as 1966 illegal abortions remained the main cause of avoidable maternal deaths (Brookes 1988). Thus, backstreet and self-induced abortions with all the risks, or enforced childbirth often resulting in poverty, continued to be the only options for working-class women confronted with an unwanted pregnancy.

Hindell and Simms (1968) argue that the ALRA initially concentrated its efforts on an educational rather than political role. However, this undervalues and misses the core of the organization's activities as it was highly political in its arguments and its aim of articulating working-class women's needs for legalized abortion. The ALRA's political activity was centred outside of Parliament, among Labour women's groups and the wider labour movement in an attempt to appeal for grass-roots support among the working class. During the 1950s the activities of ALRA declined as the original activists had either retired, suffered ill health or died. ALRA was to become the key organization in securing parliamentary reform. By this stage, however, ALRA had lost its organic connections with the broader labour and socialist movements and had become a small, middle-class lobbying organization.

The Abortion Act 1967

ALRA sponsored a number of failed Private Members Bills from 1952. In the early 1960s ALRA membership was only 200 but by 1966, the year of David Steele's Abortion Bill, it had risen to over 1,000. Although ALRA's membership was overwhelmingly middle class, they saw abortion as a social issue. Its chairwoman, Madeleine Simms, summed up the organization's attitude: 'I have to say, looking back, that the issues of public health and injustice impelled us, more than feminism or any thought of the right to choose' (Simms 1992). This was reflected both in ALRA tactics and in the parliamentary debate. ALRA commissioned and utilized opinion polls to argue its case. In the early 1960s there was a heightened public awareness of the need for medical abortion as a result of the 'thalidomide scandal' – high rates of mortality and deformations in babies as a result of thalidomide being prescribed to pregnant women. In 1962, 72 per cent of those polled supported abortion if the baby would have been born deformed (Hindell and Simms 1968).[2] ALRA members wrote to the press and assiduously lobbied MPs. David Steele's bill became law with extra government time from the Labour government, and with the help of an intake of new, well-educated, middle-class Labour MPs who also supported the legalization of homosexuality and the abolition of capital punishment. The parliamentary debate was couched in terms which indicated that abortion on demand was not part of abortion law reformers' agenda, whatever their private views were. MPs in their speeches made it clear that the law was designed to ease the lot of the minority of women who could not cope with maternity: women whose pregnancy was the result of rape, older women already worn out by childbirth, women whose life and health would be adversely affected (Sheldon 1993). The debate was entirely about how liberal the restrictions on abortion should be (Greenwood and Young 1976).

The outcome, the Abortion Act 1967, is a classic piece of reforming legislation. It allowed for lawful therapeutic abortion where two doctors judged 'that the continuation of the pregnancy would involve risk to the life of the pregnant woman or of injury to the physical or mental health of the pregnant woman or any existing children of her family greater than if the pregnancy were terminated'. It also permitted termination where there was a risk that the child would be born suffering from 'physical or mental abnormalities as to be seriously handicapped'. There was no legal time limit written into the 1967 Act but with the provisions of the Infant Life Preservation Act the time limit was 28 weeks (Issac 1994). The Act allowed provision for doctors and nurses to refuse to carry out abortions on the grounds of conscience. However, the drafting of the Act permitted medical abortion on a large scale. The wording relied on the concept of greater risk, but in fact abortion is an extremely safe medical procedure, far safer than a full-term pregnancy. In practice, therefore, a woman who wanted an abortion could have one if she could find sympathetic doctors. For the first time the majority of women had a reasonable expectation of gaining access to safe, legal abortion. The number of backstreet abortions fell dramatically but the total number of abortions rose from 35,000 in 1968 to 141,000 in 1975. While not all women could get NHS abortions, because of different funding decisions and doctors in some areas organizing around the conscience clause (the number of NHS abortions fell from 65 per cent in 1968 to only 49 per cent by 1975), the impact of the Act was none the less profound and enduring.

The underlying causes of the liberal legislation, of which the Abortion Act was a part, were rooted in longer term social changes affecting women. Women have always worked, and early capitalist development drew working-class women into the new factories and urban centres. However, the hardships of maternity meant that many women when they could, or when work was not available to them, left the labour market at childbearing. Under increasing ideological pressure it had become relatively common in the inter-war period and through to the 1950s for women to leave the workforce at marriage or at the birth of the first child. The 1961 census, however, showed a major shift in trends of women's employment. By 1961 it was apparent that large numbers of women were beginning to re-enter the labour market after a break for child-rearing, the over-35s made up the major increases in women's participation in the workforce in the 1950s and 1960s (Coyle 1988). This trend has continued up to the 1990s with fewer births, and increasingly early return to work after the birth of a child. These were significant changes; women were in the workforce in increased numbers and to stay, and increasingly they were organized.

The late 1960s and 1970s saw a series of struggles for equality for women in the workplace. The Ford women may not have achieved equal pay but their strike in 1968 was emblematic. Student unrest from 1968 onwards brought many young women into active politics either on the left or in small local women's groups. There was a tremendous sense of new-found freedom for thousands of women beyond the confines of the Women's Liberation Movement (WLM) (Clegg 1996). Many of these women were white-collar workers who became active in their trade unions raising women's demands on equal pay, child care, abortion rights, and sexual harassment in the workplace. They were the forces which would mobilize in defence of the 1967 Act as it came under attack.

The defence of the Act

From as early as 1969 there have been parliamentary attacks attempting to restrict both the circumstances in which abortion is permitted and the number of weeks when termination is legally allowable. These seeming technicalities are driven by an ideological desire to stop abortions altogether. The anti-abortionists have focused on foetal viability as a way of trying to mobilize support for their views. However, the underlying support for abortion has strengthened not weakened. Support for the Abortion Act 1967 has remained solid, based on the widespread acceptance that safe, legal abortion is the preferable option. How, and whether, this support manifested itself in action to defend the Act depended on the particular political conjuncture. This can be best demonstrated by analysing the attacks and the responses they provoked.

There were a number of early attempts to restrict abortion (Norman St John Stevens in 1969, Byant Godman Irvman in 1970, John Hunt in 1971, James White in 1972, Michael Grylls in 1973–4). Faced with the possibility that one of these attacks could succeed, the National Abortion Campaign (NAC) was set up in 1975 to defend the

Act against the James White Private Members Bill. White's bill proposed changing the grounds to make abortions more restrictive, separating referral agencies and clinics with statutory approval and making access more difficult through clinics in areas where NHS provision was inadequate (Berer 1988; German 1988). The campaign involved political activists on the revolutionary left (the International Marxist Group, International Socialists), as well as the Women's Liberation Movement, and the Communist Party. Strategy was contested within NAC nationally, but the influence of left-wing ideas including within the WLM meant that there was a concentration on workplaces and trade unions as well as on pressuring Labour MPs to oppose James White's bill. Motions defending the Act, and more generally in favour of a woman's right to choose, were supported by trade unions. Street petitions were organized. In June 1975 the NAC's first national demonstration mobilized 40,000 marchers in London, with a further 700 in Glasgow.

The next big mobilizations were against John Corrie's 1979[3] attempt to reduce the time limit from 28 to 20 weeks by only allowing abortion if there was a 'grave' risk to the life of the woman or 'substantial risk' of 'serious' injury to the mental or physical health of the woman's existing children and family. The Corrie bill also proposed widening the conscience clause and a separation of referral agencies from clinics. Corrie moreover marked the first attempt to amend the 1967 Act under the new Thatcher-led Tory government and the mobilization reflected wider anxieties among trade unionists and on the left about what the new government would do to welfare. Opinion polls showed a majority in favour of the existing abortion law. The Trade Union Congress (TUC), Labour Women and Labour Party Conferences all had strong resolutions attacking the bill. An estimated 80,000 people, many with union banners, attended national demonstrations sponsored by the TUC (Brown 1991). Unions wrote to all sponsored MPs. The British Medical Association led the medical professions' opposition to the bill. NAC formed Campaign Against Corrie (CAC) as a single-issue campaign. CAC produced twelve leaflets each with a distribution of 15,000. Large numbers of local CAC groups were formed to petition, organize and support demonstrations. The National Union of Students called for a week of action, and a CAC organized rally sponsored by the South East TUC was attended by 15–20,000 people, while on the same day 7,000 lobbied MPs.

There was also organized support for Corrie, with petitions in churches, letters to MPs, and a counter-demonstration organized by the Society for the Protection of the Unborn Child (SPUC) and LIFE with 3,000 marching to Downing Street with a wreath for the abortions following the 1967 Act. Wreaths were also distributed to the TUC and the Department of Health and Social Security with 15–18,000 attending a mass lobby of the House of Commons. There was no disguising, however, that the anti-abortion lobby was in the minority and that anti-abortionists were on the defensive. The parliamentary threat was, however, extremely serious. The bill gained 242 votes to 98 on its second reading but ran out of time and was withdrawn by Corrie.

The significance and the extent of extra-parliamentary opposition to Corrie cannot be overestimated. It stretched far beyond those who could be defined as political activists. As a result of the campaigns and activity in trade unions, access to abortion had become embedded as a basic demand which was seen to impact directly on the lives of both working-class women and men. The 1970s had seen repeated struggles over jobs, pay and conditions in the public sector, many of these struggles had been led by women. There were also strikes in support of services which provided for the health and welfare of the mass of people. This is not to suggest that there was political unity about tactics within CAC. To the contrary, there were fierce arguments even extending to who should lead the massive TUC march – trade unionists or a women-only contingent. There were also major disagreements within the women's movement, the last WLM National Conference had been held in 1978 and there has not been one since. The women's movement splintered, with many women joining the Labour Party while most radical feminists concentrated on issues of pornography and violence against women and became both more separatist and separated from other social movements (Segal 1987).

The next major threat to the Abortion Act came in David Alton's 1988 Abortion Amendment Bill, again aimed at reducing the time from 28 weeks to, initially, 18 weeks and then, in an attempt to get the bill through, to 24 weeks. The political climate when Alton introduced his bill was very different from 1975, or even from 1979. The Thatcher government had succeeded in enforcing major defeats on organized labour, and the women's movement, already fractured in 1979, was reduced to a series of competing feminisms. There had been debates within NAC leading to a split between those who saw the need for a campaigning single-issue organization, and women who wanted to expand the agenda to consider reproductive rights. The focus on reproductive rights was a reaction to the criticism that the organization's emphasis on abortion was too narrow and ignored the experience of black, ethnic minority women and poor women whose rights are curtailed through a denial of their right to bear children through enforced sterilization or the involuntary administration of long-acting contraceptive drugs (Berer 1988). As an analysis of the class nature of reproduction this view had much to recommend it. However, in practice the argument obscured the need to mobilize to defend the 1967 Act as a vital part of any attempt by women to control their fertility as opposed to having it controlled for them.

As in 1980, NAC formed Fight the Alton Bill (FAB), and a national demonstration was called co-sponsored by the TUC and the Labour Party. Support for the Act remained at very high levels all through the 1980s with 80 per cent of people, including Conservative voters, agreeing to the statement that a woman should be able to decide on abortion in consultation with her doctor. However, the general attacks on organized labour by the Thatcher government had taken their toll and the level of active mobilization was much lower than in 1979/1980. Later in 1988 there was a major defeat with the passing of the infamous Clause 28 which restricted teachers' ability to inform young people about same-sex relationships.

Alton's bill was talked out of time, but the arguments about viability had already begun to have an effect. In February 1985, for example, there was a voluntary agreement with clinics and the Minister of Health not to undertake abortions after 24 weeks unless there was a risk to the woman's health. A Department of Health and Social Security (DHSS) circular requested the same for NHS hospitals and in 1986 agreement not to perform abortions after 24 weeks became a condition of the licence. This may sound like a minor adjustment, but because doctors are cautious when estimating the number of weeks of pregnancy the effect was to make late abortion very difficult. The reasons for late abortion include lack of NHS access, older women confused by signs associated with the menopause, and younger, vulnerable women who may not be aware of, or are too afraid to tell anyone about their pregnancy.

Despite these curtailments, and despite the rhetoric, many MPs at the heart of government recognized the enormous costs associated with unlawful terminations. The medical profession were also anxious not to have doubt cast on the legality of their practice. So after the defeat of Alton's bill, and a similar failure in 1989 by Anne Widdecombe to reintroduce the bill, the government moved in 1990 to present a bill based on the Warnock Committee recommendations on Human Fertilisation and Embryology. The Human Fertilisation and Embryology Act 1990 sets a limit of 24 weeks unless there is 'grave injury' to the physical or mental health of the woman, or to avoid the birth of a 'seriously' handicapped baby. However, it permits abortion to term on the following grounds: (i) if there is a risk of grave permanent injury to the physical or mental health of the woman; (ii) where the continuance of the pregnancy involves a greater risk to life of a pregnant woman than if the pregnancy was terminated; or (iii) where there is substantial risk that the child would be born seriously handicapped. The liberal interpretation of the Abortion Act 1967 has therefore been maintained while removing any absolute time limit. This represents an enormous victory in the struggle for abortion rights. Today, three decades after the 1967 Act, abortion in Britain remains legal, and despite variations and under-funding in the NHS, largely accessible. The scourge of illegal abortion has not returned.

Abortion struggles in the United States

Abortion was legalized in the United States in 1973 through the *Roe* v. *Wade* Supreme Court decision. Before 1973, the situation was uneven but in most states abortion was illegal except when a woman's life was threatened. A woman who wanted an abortion had to appeal to a hospital committee to prove she had a need for what was defined as a therapeutic (necessary) as opposed to an elective (unnecessary) abortion. This gave the medical profession ultimate control over women's reproduction. As hospitals monitored and restricted the numbers of abortions most safe abortions were carried out privately and discreetly for middle-class women. Poor and minority women were generally excluded from municipal hospitals, although large numbers were admitted due to complications following illegal abortions (Pollack Petchesky 1986). It is estimated that at least 200,000 illegal abortions occurred annually by the late 1960s (Solinger 1998). In New York, 80 per cent of deaths caused by illegal abortions involved black and Puerto Rican women (Davies 1982).

During the 1960s women's lives changed as part of the massive expansion of the American economy. Increasing numbers of women became college and university educated, both married and unmarried women were drawn into the labour market, women were delaying marriage and childbearing and there was an increase in divorce and female-headed households. All these factors were influential in decreasing fertility rates (Pollack Petchesky 1986). As a result of these changes, 'second wave' feminism grew from the contradictions between the prevailing ideology that advocated that women's primary role was in the home, and women's real experiences outside the home (Petty *et al.* 1987).

One strand of feminism which developed was the National Organization for Women (NOW), established by Betty Friedan in 1966. The identification of what Friedan referred to as 'the problem with no name' – the futility of the lives of full-time housewives – found support among middle-class college educated women who felt psychologically and socially trapped. NOW concentrated on pursuing legal changes in education, employment and reproductive rights as a means to achieve equality with men. NOW, although often at the forefront of political struggles, was, and still is, essentially a liberal organization pressurising the state to resolve gender inequalities. It reflects and promotes the interests of its predominantly white, middle-class membership.

The other strand of the WLM developed in the late 1960s and early 1970s out of a period of social and political turbulence which saw the increasing militancy of civil rights activists, the rise of Black Power, anti-Vietnam War protests, and student movements, and in the development of an active 'New Left'. The New Left differed from the 'old' left of the 1930s Depression. The old left had been decimated by McCarthyism during the late 1940s and early 1950s and discredited by its association with Stalinism. The New Left protested against 'the system' and was 'anti-establishment', without any clear political or theoretical analysis of the exploitative social relations that the capitalist system was based on. The movement lacked coherent politics, it was influenced by a mixed bag of 'isms': anarchism, socialism, pacifism, existentialism, humanism, transcendentalism, bohemianism, populism, mysticism and black nationalism (Newfield 1967). Unlike in Britain, there were no systematic links with the labour force though the trade unions. Trade union membership is much lower in America than it is in Britain, and the Democratic Party does not have the same organic links with the trade unions as the Labour Party does with the British unions.

The two key strands of the WLM developed from a period of economic growth accompanied by changes in women's lives and heightened general political activity. In 1970 over 50,000 protesters took part in a national demonstration for free abortion on demand, no forced sterilization, 24-hour childcare and equal pay for equal work (Petty *et al.* 1987). Much of the feminist effort to secure legal abortion was, however, undertaken by litigation through the courts (Kesselman 1998). The 1973 *Roe* v. *Wade* Supreme Court ruling was based on a recognition of reproductive decision-making as an aspect of the Constitutionally enshrined right to privacy, which in turn was based on freeing individuals from unwarranted government intrusion. The decision determined that although women had the right to privacy, this right was not absolute as the state was deemed to have an increasing interest as a pregnancy progressed, justified by the notion of the viability of the foetus (Cohan 1986). Pollack Petchesky (1986) argues that abortion became legal at this time principally because it could not remain illegal, due to the wide-scale flouting of an unenforceable law, and militant and continuous pressure from the WLM whose demand for abortion became supported by the population lobby (albeit for different reasons). The role of the WLM was clearly crucial in determining the 1973 decision, but it subsequently became ineffective in its defence.

There was a distinct decline in the level of struggles from 1974 onwards as the American economy went into recession and the political climate moved to the right. Within three years, the Supreme Court decision was systematically eroded, leaving one of the most liberal abortion laws virtually inaccessible for poor and minority women (Fied 1998). The Hyde Amendment 1976 prohibited Medicaid-funded abortion except 'where the life of the mother would be endangered'. Unlike in Britain where the anti-abortion movement was a relatively defensive one, in the United States it moved into a position of attack. President Ronald Reagan began appointing anti-abortion judges to the Supreme Court, and in 1987 Randall Terry led his first attack on an abortion clinic under the name of 'rescuing' the foetus. The viciousness of the anti-abortionists in America cannot be overstated. Operation Rescue, formed in 1988, continues to maintain a campaign of harassment and violence outside abortion clinics. In 1994 two doctors and one of their assistants were murdered in two separate incidents, and another two abortion clinic employees were murdered in 1995. In a 1989 case, *Webster* v. *Reproductive Health Services*, the Supreme Court upheld a Missouri law stating that 'life begins at conception' and came within one vote of overturning *Roe* v. *Wade* which would have made abortion illegal. However, by building on *Webster* v. *Reproductive Health Services*, over 700 anti-abortion rights bills were introduced between 1989 and 1992 into state legislatures (Solinger 1998). These changes represent a major defeat for abortion rights.

The defeat can be explained partly by the shifting balance of political forces towards the right, but also lies within the nature of the WLM itself. The abortion issue in the United States is an example of a radical movement which has become increasingly reformist in its strategies and solutions. As a result of the rightward shift, the movement itself followed, preventing adequate mobilization to defend gains which came under attack. Despite the fact that minority women, alongside white women, had a need for abortion and suffered disproportionately from its illegality, minority women were not drawn into the WLM's mobilization over abortion rights. It was particularly difficult for minority women to speak out in support of birth control and abortion due to America's obsession with eugenics which re-emerged during the 1950s and 1960s in the form of population 'explosion' theories. The preferred method of family planning for the poor by the American government has consistently been sterilization as this offers a long-term and permanent solution to population control (Pollack Petchesky 1986). Between 1907 and 1940 many states passed eugenic laws that allowed involuntary sterilization of the 'socially inadequate', those with hereditary disorders and physical disability. These laws, which in some states remain on the statute books, mainly affected the mentally ill and poor black and Hispanic women (Ginsburg 1992). The forced sterilization of minority women has become a consistent policy and often made a condition of obtaining an abortion for women dependent on Aid for Dependent Children (AFDC).

For minority women the issue of reproduction was centred around women having control, and the material means and access to services and resources to be able to make real choices. For poor women abortion historically is the result of desperate material conditions rather than exclusively a desire to limit births (Davies 1982). The WLM failed to appeal to minority women as their focus on abortion rights was too narrow, excluding the right to have children and to raise them with sufficient material resources and support. These associated issues surrounding reproduction, health and child rearing were not taken up by the WLM, leading to its isolation from working-class minority and white women. Therefore, when black women did start to organize in the early 1970s, they had a wider focus than abortion rights and demanded voluntary control, not forced control (Ross 1998). By the 1980s groups like the National Black Women's Health Project broadened their demands further by making links between reproductive control and such issues as paid parental leave, child care provision, welfare expansion, decent housing and demands for a living wage (Brenner 1993).

The first attack (the Hyde Amendment in 1976) which principally affected poor women received little response from the WLM, who, between 1977 and 1982 concentrated its efforts instead towards achieving ratification of the Equal Rights Amendment (ERA). The WLM mistakenly felt secure in the fact that it had successfully won a victory with the 1973 ruling and therefore turned its attention elsewhere. This lack of organized response to abortion attacks paved the way for the 1989 case, *Webster* v. *Reproductive Health Services*. In stark contrast to the response to previous attacks this decision increased the mobilization of the WLM. The reason for this was founded on the fact that the 1989 ruling came close to overturning the principle of abortion rights.

Pollack Petchesky (1986) points out that poor women do continue to obtain abortions, but under extremely difficult conditions. This is because those states that provide Medicaid funding are geographically concentrated, and changes in law have only applied in some states. But by 1995 only 13 per cent of abortions were paid for using public funds and by early 1996 only seventeen states covered abortion for health reasons, and ten of these are likely to change their stand (Fied 1998). The bulk of working-class women have to travel to accommodating states, and are forced to meet the costs through borrowing and/or diverting money away from other essential expenditures such as rent and food. At abortion clinics women are frequently confronted by blockades, protests and bomb threats from anti-abortion groups who violently fight to overturn abortion rights by targeting the weakest and least defended component: access to services.

These defeats have catastrophic consequences. They do not, however, mean that anti-abortion measures have popular support or that the right have won the argument. The 'silent majority' still support abortion: in a poll of African-Americans this support was 83 per cent in 1991 (Ross 1998). This is not surprising, since for the majority of working-class women access to abortion remains vital. Abortion in America is not illegal but its curtailment represents a worsening of the lives of women. The underlying rationale and the long-term social changes that underpinned *Roe* v. *Wade* remain, but the outcome of the struggle will depend on organization and mobilization by the pro-choice movement.

Conclusion

We have argued that abortion is a class issue in two senses. Access to abortion is dependent on class position, and political mobilization in struggles for abortion rights is based in class issues. We are not arguing that reform can only come about if the struggle for abortion involves the broader labour movement and working-class women, both black and white. The passage of the 1967 Act clearly demonstrates that this is not so. Where there are broader social and economic changes underpinning reform liberal pressure groups can be extremely effective. This was the case in the 1960s when the medical and liberal establishments correctly diagnosed that the changes in women's lives meant that safe and effective fertility control was becoming an urgent social issue. However, the successful defence of abortion rights was based on the movement's roots in the working-class movement. The conditions were not the same in America. Despite the brave and concerted efforts by many women in the WLM and beyond, activists have not been able to defend abortion rights. Major attacks from the right have undermined access to abortion. One of the principal failures of the American pro-abortion movement has been the inability to involve minority and working-class women who are most directly affected by the attacks. There are some grounds for optimism in the recent involvement of women of colour in mobilizations (Ross 1998). However, whether the pro-choice movement succeeds in moving forward will depend on a politics which can fight to restore Medicaid and health benefits for all.

We have also argued that the broader changes in women's lives, which have drawn more women into paid employment, have provided the structural basis for popular support for abortion rights. Again this is not an argument for crude determination of the political by the economic. Our comparison between Britain and the United States has shown that broadly similar social structural changes can, under different political circumstances, produce very different outcomes. Any analysis, therefore, needs to take into account the balance of political forces. The underlying structural changes are, however, important in understanding the support for abortion reform in popular consciousness. They explain why despite the strength of the political right in America there is a deep ambivalence among legislatures to the total re-criminalization of abortion.

Abortion rights have been at the centre of struggles for women's equality and social and economic freedom for the last three decades. The reason is not hard to find. Women will always choose abortion when personal circumstances mean it that is their best or only option, but criminalized and semi-legal abortion meant untold misery for hundreds of thousands of women. Control of fertility is central to women's health and welfare, and their social and political rights. We remain convinced that abortion rights, 'a woman's right to choose' both 'free' and 'on demand' abortions, are fundamental to women's lives and well-being. Historical analysis shows the importance of remembering, but as well as remembering we believe it is important to contribute to history as actors. For us, therefore, abortion rights remain a question of practical politics.

Notes

1   It was not until 1967 that contraception became freely available in Britain with the Family Planning Act.
2   Using arguments about deformity became the subject of bitter argument in later debates with people with disabilities. At the time, however, ALRA used the Thalidomide scandal to shock people into the realization of the consequences of lack of abortion options.
3   Between White and Corrie there had been a further two attempts to restrict abortion; first by William Benyon in 1977 and then by Bernard Braine in 1978. The Labour Party had attempted to defuse the controversy by holding discussions with both pro- and anti-abortion groups.

10 Riots and urban unrest in Britain in the 1980s and 1990s

A critique of dominant explanations[1]

Rumy Hasan

Introduction

The riots and social unrest which took place in several British cities during the 1980s and 1990s marked a watershed in British history in that the chief protagonists involved were, in the main, Afro-Caribbean and Asian youth born or brought up in Britain. Unlike many of their parents, they were no longer prepared to tolerate quietly systematic discrimination and poor socio-economic conditions – centring on low-skill and poorly paid jobs, sub-standard housing and low levels of education – all buttressed by endemic racism. This was tantamount to a vociferous, angry, and frequently violent rejection of being treated as 'second class citizens'. The magnitude of the unrest had, arguably, at least one significant political impact on the British establishment: a recognition that there was in the urban centres a large and growing black population which was here to stay. And in recognition of this, the epithet 'Black British' largely replaced the pejorative description 'immigrants'. However, as will be seen, the riots and disturbances were not solely confined to young blacks but involved a substantial number of white youths as well.

The legal definition of what constitutes a riot has altered over the last decade, but the 1980s and 1990s saw repeated disturbances in a number of towns and cities. The most significant were those in Bristol in 1980, in London, Liverpool, Manchester and various others towns in 1981, in Birmingham, Bristol, London, Liverpool and various other towns in 1985, in Cardiff, Tyneside and Oxford in 1991, and in Bradford in 1995. These were serious confrontations that shed light upon how society itself is structured. They have also motivated considerable study from a plethora of sources: governments and other state institutions, political parties, academic researchers and community groups. For this reason, this chapter is different to others in this collection. Riots have not been 'hidden from (recent) history', indeed they have been the subject of much debate. Here the aim is to critically examine the debates regarding the motives for, and nature of, riots and unrest, before concluding with a brief examination of their impact.

Interpretations and explanations

Providing a list of theoretical explanations of riots can be problematic. The categories can range widely covering different conventional academic disciplines. Here I look at those broadly distinct theories that are primarily located in differing political ideologies, examining, where appropriate, other 'non-political' theories that may underpin them. The following are examined: conservative, liberal (in Britain, usually taken to mean social democratic as well), black nationalist and Marxist. This cross-section is different to those normally found in the literature. Thus, though blacks feature prominently in British riots, the black nationalist view – which, at the very least, examines riots from a black perspective – is rarely accredited in discussions of riots (see, for example, Taylor 1984; Benyon and Solomos 1987; Waddington 1992). Marxist explanations when discussed, are invariably located within a wider set of ideas, usually termed 'radical'. Lea and Young (1982) omit even discussing the radical view; merely confining themselves to conservative and liberal theses.

Conservative explanations

For those on the right of the Conservative Party (such as Enoch Powell and Margaret Thatcher), one key factor that provides the explanation of recurring riots during the modern-day period is the presence of large black migrant communities in the inner cities. This thesis is corroborated by, on the one hand, the preponderance of blacks in riots, and on the other, with the absence of riots in those cities which have a low percentage of black residents, such as Glasgow (Lea and Young 1992: 5) (though it needs pointing out that Glasgow has a fairly large Asian community). The infamous assertion by Margaret Thatcher in 1978 about the possibility of Britain being 'swamped by people with a different culture' (Barker 1981: 15) can be viewed as providing a classic right-wing explanation for riotous behaviour. The supposed 'different culture' is used to explain the inability of black migrants to cope with periods of relative hardship such as the rapidly rising level of unemployment in the first half of the

1980s. For the extreme right (including Nazi sympathizers), the solution is obvious: the systematic repatriation of blacks (meaning all non-whites). This was Enoch Powell's clarion call in the 1960s – and he continued to advocate it thereafter. Thus, he warned that the 1981 riots were only the beginning of further racial problems (*Sunday Telegraph*, 9 May 1982), later arguing for the government to repatriate 'immigrants' to avoid 'a Britain unimaginably wracked by dissension and violent disorder' (*Financial Times*, 2 September 1985). In a similar vein, the right-wing Tory MP Harvey Proctor called for a ban on black 'commonwealth immigration' after the 1985 riots (*Daily Telegraph*, 8 October 1985).

However, it is probably true to say that mainstream Conservative politicians have been reluctant to play the 'race card' with regard to riots which, as argued earlier, is a consequence of their gradual acceptance – albeit in many cases reluctantly – of 'Black Britons' being a legitimate section of the population. Rather, for them and conservatives in general, riots are viewed as a law and order problem, as criminal acts which must be treated accordingly. The former Conservative Home Secretary, Douglas Hurd, put this view bluntly after the 1985 Handsworth riots in Birmingham: 'it is not a case history for sociologists to pore over, but a case for the police' (*Guardian*, 23 September 1985). The prescription flowing from this is firm policing and, consequently, an unstinting support for the police – even when they are so often accused of being the instigator of riots. The logic underpinning this belief is clear: laws are made by demo-cratically-elected governments and as such, must be adhered to by all concerned. Riots and disorder represent clear breaches of the law and therefore cannot, and must not, be tolerated. It is the duty of the police to ensure that all such breaches are quickly suppressed – hence the emphasis on effective policing methods. As a corollary to this, social and economic matters are not given much importance – for to do so would be to attribute at least a portion of blame to the government itself. The polity is considered sufficiently flexible to fulfil the needs of all, including those with genuine grievances. Democratic institutions provide a satisfactory channel for addressing any such grievances, and only through these is it legitimate to press for change.

In so far as the cause of riots is concerned there is, in conservative thought, frequently the recourse to conspiracy theories (Kettle and Hodges 1982: 20) whereby 'external influences' or 'outside agitators' are key players. It is certainly a particular favourite of the popular press. This assumes, in essence, that the 'masses' are gullible; a fact that enables external agents (that is, political activists or agitators) to act out their conspiracy by inciting crowds to riot. The origins of this view go back at least to a group of late nineteenth-century conservative theorists (Tarde, Sighele and Le Bon) described by Rule (1988: 91) as 'irrationalists' who were attempting to make sense of an increasing trend of social disorder in the aftermath of the Paris commune in 1871. For these theorists, this destructive tendency was irrational or deviant in comparison with the calm orderliness of everyday normality. The irrational behaviour, they argued, stems from being actively part of a group, or more specifically, a crowd. Le Bon put it clearly:

> by the mere fact that he forms part of an organised crowd, a man descends several rungs in the ladder of civilisation. ... He possesses the spontaneity, the violence, the ferocity, and also the enthusiasm and heroism of primitive beings ... and [can] be induced to commit acts contrary to his most obvious interests and best-known habits.
> (Le Bon 1903: 36)

It follows, therefore, that gatherings, assemblies and crowds will have a tendency to lead to irrational, counter-productive, behaviour 'against' the interests of individuals that form them. Moreover, the lapse into irrationality presents the conspirator with the opportunity of injecting damaging ideas and actions on the masses. Being part of a crowd causes a radical (meaning in this sense worsening) change in an individual's consciousness. However, it should be noted that though this analysis is intended to have universal applicability, it is particularly targeted at those whom Le Bon perceives to be of 'inferior forms of evolution' – such as 'women, savages, and children' (1903: 40). The trigger for the formation of the crowd in the first place is also rooted in consciousness – as Sighele puts it: 'the display of an emotional state touches off the same state in he who witnesses it' (quoted in Rule 1988: 94). But, because one does not have to be a direct witness, we can see how this analysis can also be used to explain a common occurrence of modern urban unrest in an age of mass telecommunications, that of 'copycat' or 'contagious' riots, where riots spread like wildfire from city to city after the participants view the events on television or hear about them on the radio.

The conservative explanations suffer from fundamental weaknesses. First, it is not made clear, nor proven how, conspirators are able to bring significant numbers of people out on the streets with the set aim of rioting (as opposed to other forms of demonstrations) – there is no evidence, for example, of systematic word of mouth operations, leafleting or flyposting that might indicate a conspiracy is being planned. Second, there is poor empirical evidence for the very existence of conspirators (Kettle and Hodges 1982); rather than these being instrumental in causing riots (in contrast to demonstrations and campaigns), agitators tend to join in once a riot is underway, for it is precisely in these circumstances that they hope their ideas will have a greater hearing and consonance with those involved. Thus the conservative theory fails to explain the dynamics (that is, the 'how' and 'why') of crowd formation – a prerequisite to full-blooded riots, be these autonomous or induced by conspirators. It might be suggested that the existence of an emotional state provides this. But it is not clear what precisely triggers the emotional state in the first instance that engenders crowd formation. Plainly, this must be a source that conveys a similar emotional response in a group of people – the precursor to crowd formation and riotous behaviour. However, this begs the question: where does the source itself originate? Here we arrive at a key limitation of conservative theories: the absence of locating satisfactory sources for the start of the process that leads to rioting. This leaves the analysis exposed, regardless of whether the subsequent explication of the riot process is rooted in reality. Thus conservative explanations suffer from an important lacuna in explaining the triggering mechanism. Viewing riots as a law and order issue results in focusing on effects and ignoring the underlying causes.

Liberal / social-democratic explanations

In sharp contrast to conservative theories, liberal/social-democratic explanations do acknowledge socio-economic and political factors in explaining underlying causes of riotous behaviour.[2] The liberal/social-democratic thesis contends that there is a direct causal link between social injustice and deprivation and social disturbance, that rests on firm empirical evidence which indubitably shows urban riots tending to arise in deprived localities. From this general proposition, specific socio-economic factors that encompass deprivation are located. Of these, the most important are unemployment, inadequate housing, education, and poor social amenities. Racism is acknowledged as a key factor accentuating deprivation. A confluence of adverse factors prepares the ground upon which crime becomes endemic and social ferment can take hold: an egregious incident (such as a perceived act of injustice) may then trigger the potential for disturbance in becoming an actual disturbance, which in some instances translates into a full-blown riot.

In locating the root causes of the potential to riot, analysis focuses on why conditions have so deteriorated and what can be done to alleviate them. It therefore follows that the emphasis shifts on to the various policies of government, in combination with the institutional mechanisms that underpin them – for clearly these have, at least for the localities or communities concerned, failed to provide the necessary structures and wherewithal to ensure some degree of social harmony. The prescription flowing from this is for changes in government policy to enable the channelling of resources to deprived communities to alleviate the root problems; together with greater efforts to incorporate deprived groups into the polity. A corollary is the need for more 'sensitive policing', implying a recognition of, and the shift away from confrontational methods towards 'community policing', but the police are always given full support and their role or legitimacy in society remains unquestioned.

How precisely does deprivation lead to riots? Benyon (1987) notes that emphasis should be laid on *relative* deprivation and unrealized expectations where unrealized expectations lead to a build-up in frustration or dissonance that can find expression in aggressive behaviour. Relative deprivation theories, however, are subject to an obvious and fundamental criticism. If frustration or dissonance is the precondition for dissatisfaction with the prevailing state of affairs – to be possibly triggered off by some stimulus into aggressive behaviour – then equally, dissatisfaction and aggressive behaviour must surely imply the existence of frustration or dissonance. If so, the two assertions are merely equivalents and, therefore, it appears that these theories suffer from circularity, and hence lack explanatory power. They might, however, provide a useful insight if they could provide guidelines as to at what point or level frustration triggers off aggression, though there remain problems of measurement – for Aya (1979: 66) suggests these are merely 'speculative projections' on social conditions and patterns of change; an assertion supported by the fact that empirical evidence providing such critical levels is weak (Rule 1988: 213–23). Rather, Aya insists that 'volcanic theories' such as relative deprivation and frustration suffer from three fallacies: first, their lack of political focus on state institutions; second, they 'never identify specific power groups acting politically to advance and defend their interests'; and third, their failure to explain the route from social change to grievances, and from grievances to revolt, so that 'grievances may "motivate" rebellion, but they do not explain it'.

In sum, therefore, we may suggest that liberal/social-democratic theories either ignore or underplay the politics of riots – like conservative explanations – viewing them essentially as irrational acts. The recognition of socio-economic factors, though a step forward, still does not, in and of itself, provide a valid explanation of how socio-economic discontent can give rise to riotous behaviour at certain junctures. Moreover, the liberal/social-democratic critique of the socio-economic and political arrangement is limited to not only accepting but defending it in its fundamentals; and in this way it also parallels conservative theories.

A view that combines both conservative and liberal/social-democratic approaches is that of Campbell's feminist thesis. She argues that men – especially the unemployed – can be considered an 'inferior form' as she asserts that crime, including the partaking in 'unjustified' riots, is a 'phenomenon of masculinity' (1993: 211). Unemployed men are berated in particular for their inadequacies: absence from housework, even though they are (forcibly) 'domesticated'; 'flight from fatherhood' and their inability to take care of themselves (ibid.: 202). Though the decline of the economy and concomitant rise in unemployment is acknowledged, this is not – with respect to men – invoked for explanatory purposes, as it is by non-conservative theories discussed below. The 1991 riots in Cardiff, Oxford, and Tyneside of which Campbell writes are, in her view, simply not justified: 'these riots lacked the one thing that legitimises lawlessness: a just cause'. In stark contrast, women are treated with great sympathy: 'The political system's culpability for the catastrophes of 1991 [the riots]: it did not know how to support the women and it did not know how to challenge the men' (203). She continues, 'Crime and coercion are sustained by men. Solidarity and self-help are sustained by women. It is as stark as that' (319). In contrast, in their study of riots in 1991–92, Power and Tunstall – while also pointing to the fact that the rioters were almost entirely young men – nonetheless stress the importance of socio-economic conditions in instilling riotous behaviour: 'lack of work, lack of direction, lack of role and lack of independence led to a pointless existence for many young men' (1997: 43).

'Black nationalist' explanations

As with the preceding explanations, what may be described as 'black nationalist' explanations vary in their emphases, so we shall try and distil the key elements which comprise them. The term gained prominence in America during the 1960s at the height of the Black Power movement and acted as a significant counterpoint, both theoretically and politically, to the more mainstream civil rights movement. At its core is the emphasis on race – specifically, the racial oppression of black (that is, non-white) people. It therefore follows that racism is fundamental to explaining the dynamic behind black people's attempts to achieve social justice and liberation. In terms of political organization and strategy, some degree of separatism (meaning 'black-only') is advocated. Consequently, the focus of analysis tends to be almost entirely on black people, and how they relate to the 'white power structures' in a deeply racist society. A cornerstone of discourse is the hostile relationship between the police and black youths. Black nationalists share with the liberal/social-democratic view the importance of socio-economic factors in explaining the dynamic of black unrest; indeed these are invariably assumed, without need for explicit analysis. But, unlike the liberals, they assert that racism is so imbued in society that 'institutional racism' is the norm, and it is this which is responsible for the racial oppression and deprivation of black people. This was clearly expressed in an editorial of a special double issue of *Race and Class*: 'to allege that unemployment or social deprivation is the cause of the "riots" is to pretend that racism is not also the cause of unemployment and deprivation – among blacks' (*Race and Class*, nos. 2/3, 1981–82). The impetus, then, towards riotous behaviour is firmly set against this socio-economic and political background. (It should be noted that almost all writers professing the black nationalist view abjure the use of the term 'riot' – when used, it is invariably enclosed in inverted commas – preferring instead 'rebellion' or 'insurrection'.)

Though little detailed theorizing is provided as to precisely how riots arise, it has been briefly described by, for example, Sivanandan for the 1981 riots:

> the youth of the benighted inner cities, black and white ... came together again, not so much in joint struggle as in a blinding moment of spontaneous insurrection against the impossibility of their condition.
>
> (Sivanandan 1990: 89)

Here, an acknowledgement is made of the multiracial aspect of the riots, but an important coda is later attached: 'but the blacks, by virtue of their racial oppression, were the insurrectionary tinder'. A distinguishing feature is the belief that inner cities are now 'peopled largely by a black "underclass" ' (ibid. 1990: 132). The constituents of this underclass are:

> homeworkers and sweatshop workers, casual and part-time work-
> ers, ad hoc and temporary workers, thrown up by the putting-out
> system in retailing, the flexi-system in manufacturing, and the hire
> and fire system in the expanding service sector, and among refu-
> gees, migrants, asylum-seekers.
>
> (Sivanandan 1990: 52)

Though somewhat contradictorily, Sivanandan later refers to the 'never-employed underclass' (1990: 137), and the expression 'never-employed' is also used elsewhere to describe black (and white) inner-city youth (Sivanandan 1981/2: 150). These combine to form the 'organic communities of resistance' and provide a political culture, material self-help and solidarity to cope with, and defend themselves, against an oppressive and all-too-frequent, repressive, system.[3]

Gilroy has argued that the role of community for blacks is some-how different to that of white working-class communities, suggesting that it is fundamental to explaining the dynamic of resistance to, and struggle against, racial oppression:

> localised struggles over education, racist violence and police prac-
> tices continually reveal how black people have made use of no-
> tions of community to provide the axis along which to organise
> themselves. ... The notion of community is also important for the
> way it can be used to re-establish the unity of black people in
> answer to the divisions which state policy, race relations sociology
> and common-sense racism have visited on their experience of
> domination.
>
> (Gilroy 1981/2: 212–13)

Two critical points can be made here. First, is there really a funda-mental difference between the nature/role of community when blacks are in struggle in comparison with their white counterparts? Elsewhere, Gilroy makes the tentative suggestion that:

> the counter-cultures and sub-cultures of black Britain may have
> held the movement together at certain crucial moments. They
> provide, among other things, important rituals which allow its

affiliates to recognize each other and celebrate their coming together.

(Gilroy 1987: 223)

But this is not a sufficiently convincing explanation of 'fundamental difference'. There is, after all, a long history of community involvement and support, including the 'coming and holding the movement together' in Britain during urban struggles – not least the historic and heroic role of mining communities during the strike of 1984–85 (see, for example, Charlesworth *et al.* 1996). Bohstedt, writing about riots in Devon between 1790 and 1810, argues that direct action was supported by 'horizontal and vertical networks of relationship with communities which had their own traditions (cited in Thompson 1991: 292). True, the struggle against racial oppression is a relatively novel one (though other migrants such as the Irish and Jews have also in the past had to contend with racial oppression), but it is not made clear precisely how black community involvement is radically different. Indubitably, the form of resistance expressed within black communities is often new and different – such as in music, dress, manner of speech, hairstyle, etc. – and indeed has much influenced white urban communities, but again this does not imply a key dissimilarity in the resolve and effectiveness to struggle against social injustice. Second, we need to make clear that the term 'black community' is ascribed a homogeneity that is tenuous in reality. It ignores class, religious and ethnic differences whose dynamic can be, instead of solidarity and unity, one of disunity. Granted that the majority of inner-city black communities comprise a similar socio-economic status (that is, working class – see Table 10.1), but religious and ethnic differences certainly can, and often do, lead to reactionary and divisive tensions. This, for instance, has clearly been the case between Hindus, Sikhs and Muslims in recent years, an outcome no doubt from the influence of communalist politics now so prevalent in the Indian subcontinent; and even within a nominally homogeneous ethnic or religious grouping. As the Bradford Commission's Report of the Bradford riots of 1995 points out, the use of the word community 'obscures differences within an identical community, notably those of gender and of class, and fails to recognise the range of opinions held in a "community" ' (1996: 92). The Report cites the case of an Asian man defining his communities thus: 'I would view myself as a member of the following communities, depending on the context and in no particular order: Black, Asian, Azad Kashmiri, Kashmiri, Mirpuri, Jat, Maril'ail, Kungriwalay, Pakistani, English, British, Yorkshireman, Bradfordian, from

Bradford Moor', and then goes on to state: 'I could use the term "community" in any of these contexts and it would have meaning. Any attempt to divide me only as one of these would be meaningless'.

Indeed, to all intents and purposes, the end of the 1980s also saw the end of the political – and unifying – usage of the epithet 'black' – to be replaced by 'black' (for Afro-Caribbean) and 'Asian' (for people whose origins lie in the Indian subcontinent); not least because of the refusal by many Asians to be described as black. From this, one can conclude that, though racial oppression is key to explaining black people's propensity to resist and riot, it is by no means valid to adjunct on to this the notion that the black community *per se* provides a vital new insight to understanding the process of riotous behaviour.

The repressive element of the state confronts blacks in the shape of the police, so it is not surprising that the leitmotif of the black youths' condition is police harassment and brutality – and their resistance to it, which, on occasion, leads to a major conflagration in the form of a riot. Thus, with respect to the Bristol riot of 1980, Ramdin (1987: 503) argues that given the increase in state authoritarianism, it could actually have taken place at any time in the previous decade – in other words, all the necessary conditions had already been in place for a very long period, and so it was a riot (as, presumably, all the others were) waiting to happen. Similarly, Bhavnani *et al.* (1986: 63) point to a history of conflict in Birmingham between 'an ill disciplined and brutal force' and the black community going back to the 1960s, provoked in particular by police 'stop and search' powers. Bunyan, too, adopts this approach by insisting that it was 'years of aggressive policing' that formed the immediate cause of the 1981 riots, and moreover, this signalled the 'price of Britain's economic and social decline' (1981/2: 154).

In explaining causes of riots and prescriptions for their elimination, the black nationalist perspective combines elements of both liberal/social-democratic and Marxist views. In its unrelenting hostility to institutional racism, oppression and state repression, it largely concurs with the Marxist explanation. Both sides agree that the struggle against social injustice is endemic and inevitable in modern capitalist society. But black nationalists rarely take the analysis to its logical, revolutionary conclusion, so that, ultimately, there is a 'pulling back' to social-democratic solutions. For example, this was the case of the Report of the Review Panel, sponsored by the West Midlands County Council, following the Handsworth riots in Birmingham in 1985. All the authors of the Report (Bhavnani *et al.* 1986) – whose aim it was to provide an explicitly black perspective on the riots – were black. The

Report is a scathing indictment of the racist and oppressive nature of British society and points to the failings of social democracy but, as Gaffney (1987: 67) points out, does not fully commit itself to the rebellious strategy of challenging the system – though it must be stressed that unlike the liberal/social-democratic view, the system's fundamentals (in particular, the institutional arrangements of the state) are by no means accepted nor defended.

Thus, because the black nationalist view does not realistically foresee a revolutionary transformation of society, it parallels the liberal/social-democratic critique of institutions, and so, either explicitly or implicitly, looks to reform of the polity and the redistribution of resources in the present system as the only feasible alternative. This was precisely what was offered by the Review Panel as can be seen by their concluding summary:

> It is the main spending programmes of Government local authorities and other public agencies that must be the primary concerns of poor people in the inner cities. Community involvement and participation must embrace all of the 'usually excluded' group of people in a realistic partnership to ensure that services, facilities, jobs and resources intended for them do actually reach them.
>
> (Bhavnani *et al.* 1986: 89)

In the final analysis, therefore, the black nationalist critique of social democrats and liberals essentially amounts to their betrayal of their own, that is social-democratic, ideals. This ambivalence, however, reveals the weakness of the black nationalist position, and leaves it open to critique: if racism is so deeply embedded within the totality of modern social relations, then abolishing racism must surely be part of a process of transforming and overturning capitalism itself. Social democratic solutions will not be sufficient to transform the racist, oppressive structures of society, and in turn, stop black resistance and rebellion which they generate.

Sivanandan (1990: 57) does assert that the resistance of black communities is in essence about the overthrow of capitalism, but then does not defend this assertion, nor proceed to show how this goal might arise. Even if it were avowedly so, this would beg the obvious question of agency: are black or black-led inner-city riots (or rebellions) sufficiently powerful to overthrow the capitalist system? Given that in Britain, blacks only comprise about 5.5 per cent of the population (1991 Census), and not all are concentrated in inner cities, one would have to conclude not. Even a black population, revolutionary in consciousness, united in its determination to overthrow a system that so oppresses them, simply does not possess the power to do so *on its own*.

There are other weaknesses in the analysis. The first is the diminution of the role of the majority white population with regard to riots. Unlike the American riots of the 1960s, there is incontrovertible evidence that the British riots of the 1980s and 1990s were multiracial (Harman, 1981; Scarman 1981; Kettle and Hodges; 1982, Keith 1993) – and black nationalists generally accept this fact, but none the less give little attention to white rioters: usually a simple acknowledgement that white youths too are deprived and suffer from loss of hope. Emphasis firmly remains on black youths and the black community, with little analysis of the rebellious potential of inner-city whites and of the forging of unity between the two communities, especially during periods of urban struggles. Paradoxically, however, the post-1981 riot issue of *Race and Class* (1981/82: 245–50) itself showed that Britain (England) has a long history of riots – cataloguing some of the most important ones since 1381. Moreover, in the present period, there have also been instances of riots taking place in areas with relatively few blacks. Thus Power and Tunstall (1997: ix) show that of thirteen riots that took place in 1991 and 1992, only one involved significant numbers of minority ethnic community members. This negates the thesis put forward, as noted earlier, by some conservatives of an absence of riots in areas that are almost entirely white. But, it also counters the black nationalist view of black youth providing the 'insurrectionary tinder' for, clearly, riots occur in the absence of blacks and racial oppression.

A second weakness is the suggestion that the inner cities are now peopled largely by an inner-city black underclass. This is subject to criticism both on the grounds of population statistics and on the use of the term 'underclass' (for a discussion of the latter, see the next section). First, the 1991 Census shows that London has almost half (45 per cent) the total number of black people (again, taken to mean non-whites) in Britain, but no London borough has a majority black population. The highest proportions are in Brent (45 per cent), Newham (42 per cent), Hackney (36 per cent), Tower Hamlets (36 per cent) and Haringey (33 per cent) (1991 Census: Table A, 830). It is true that certain localities in the major cities do have majority black populations – usually some wards or groups of roads and/or blocks within larger boroughs (such as Brixton in London or Handsworth in Birmingham) – but these cannot be generalized as the totality of inner cities *per se*. The fact remains that unlike in American inner cities, blacks in British cities are still in the minority. There are no 'black-only' ghettos – indeed it is a positive sign that in comparison with America, British cities remain relatively mixed. An important implication of this is that when a major bout of unrest occurs, there is every likelihood of it encompassing both blacks and whites.

In order to test the validity of the 'underclass' thesis, we need to examine census figures. Unfortunately, the 1981 Census did not categorize citizens' 'ethnicity', so we have to refer to the 1991 Census. We may, however, make the (reasonable) assumption that the figures did not radically alter over this decade. Table 10.1 shows the socio-economic status of blacks in five inner-London boroughs with the highest concentration of black people.

Table 10.1:   Socio-economic status of non-whites in five inner-London boroughs, 1991 (in per cent)

Socio-economic group	Hackney	Haringey	Lambeth	Newham	Tower Hamlets
Employers and managers	6	8	8	8	5
Professional workers	2	3	3	3	2
Intermediate non-manual workers	10	12	11	8	11
Junior non-manual workers	16	17	20	18	12
Manual workers	11	13	11	15	9
Personal service and semi-skilled manual workers	16	15	14	18	24
Unskilled manual workers	7	5	6	4	5
Farmers and agricultural workers	1	—	—	—	—
Armed forces and miscellaneous	3	2	3	1	4
Unemployed	29	25	25	25	28

Source: *1991 Census County Report: Inner London*, Part 1, volume 1, Table 9, and Part 2, Table 93 (London: HMSO, 1993)

Note: Brent is excluded as it is not an inner-London borough.

The picture presented here does not accord well with the 'underclass thesis'. A small, though significant, proportion of blacks comprise traditional middle-class status, and an even greater comprise the skilled working class, with large numbers occupying various semi-skilled and unskilled working-class jobs. The numbers of black unemployed are high, but again it is not the majority experience. Plainly, the hard data rejects the existence of a black underclass dominating Britain's inner cities.

Marxist explanations

The starting point for a Marxist explanation of riotous behaviour is a materialist analysis of the conditions prevailing in society. In class societies, the fundamental explanatory factor of social behaviour relates to class divisions and the inevitable class struggle this generates. It therefore follows that manifestations of social unrest have their ultimate roots in class tensions so that riots/rebellions are expressions of class struggle, even when they have race, religion or ethnicity as a critical, and sometimes dominant, factor. To express it in other terms, riots and urban unrest are an expected outcome of the class struggle under certain conditions. It is these 'conditions' that need to be concretely examined to ascertain the likelihood of riotous behaviour.

The fullest empirical examination of the social conditions in the context of modern urban riots was undertaken by the Kerner Commission in the United States in 1967/68, following the major outbreak of riots in the summer of 1967. Not surprisingly, this was overwhelmingly made up of 'establishment' figures. However, the methodology and findings were remarkably materialist (including detailing the history of blacks in America since slavery), and indeed, by and large, were antithetical to the conservative viewpoint most of the Commission members no doubt held. From its study, the Commission arrived at a 'chain' in the disorders that culminated in the outbreak of riots:

> discrimination, prejudice, disadvantaged conditions, intense and pervasive grievances, a sense of tension-heightening incidents, all culminating in the eruption of social disorder at the hands of youthful, politically-aware activists.
>
> (Kerner 1968: 112)

It was pointed out that these were 'central trends' but 'not an explanation of all aspects of riots or of all rioters'. Elsewhere the Report stated that:

> while the civil disorders of 1967 were racial in character, they were not inter-racial. The 1967 disorders, as well as earlier disorders of the recent period, involved action within [black] neighbourhoods against symbols of white American society – authority and property – rather than against white people.
>
> (Kerner 1968: 110)

Though drawing very different conclusions, Marxists would broadly agree with this analysis. A similar 'chain of causality' could be provided with respect to British riots, with the important proviso that whereas in America the riots had been almost entirely black, in Britain, the major riots were multiracial. But there are irreconcilable differences in the analysis. The Kerner Report was decidedly liberal/social-democratic in its conclusions, arguing for key reforms of American institutions, channelling of significant resources to the ghettos, and calling for a radical change in white American attitudes (Kerner 1968: Chapter 17). But it never seriously questioned or challenged the fundamentals of the polity that created the appalling problems in the first place. Though the Report's conclusion were explosive. It stated that:

> what white Americans have never fully understood – but what [blacks] can never forget – is that white society is deeply implicated in the ghetto. White institutions created it, white institutions maintain it, and white society condones it.
>
> (Kerner 1968: 2)

But, of course, it did not consider the solution of a thoroughgoing transformation of society, as a Marxist reading of this would have done.

The Marxist emphasis on laying the ultimate responsibility of social unrest with the creators of the social conditions which spawn them – the ruling class – is also underplayed by both the social-democratic and the black nationalist perspectives. Moreover, as noted in the previous section, there is also the tendency in the latter to gloss over class divisions within black communities. Evidence shows that rioters as a rule, almost in their entirety, comprise the working class –

including its unemployed component (Kerner 1968; Scarman, 1981; Bradford Commission 1996). This would not be a problem for the black nationalist argument if it were the case that all blacks were part of the working class, but it is a problem when a section of the black community is not, and, instead, is part of the middle class – for evidence also shows that very few rioters hail from the middle class: this being as true for black rioters as much as it is for white. On the contrary, those hailing from the middle class often prove to be 'counter-rioters', that is, those who in the midst of a riot argue against riotous behaviour by trying to 'cool things down', as with case of the American riots analysed by the Kerner Commission (1968: 129). This, while weakening the black nationalist case, obviously strengthens Marxist class analysis.

It was noted in the previous section that Sivanandan suggests that blacks in inner cities comprise an 'underclass'. This appears to be an attempt to distance the analysis from the Marxist one which stresses the unity of working-class interests. By positing the term underclass, there is the suggestion that this is a separate 'peripheral' sub-class with interests distinct from the 'core' working class – which is predominantly white and relatively privileged. But from the Marxist perspective, the term 'underclass' is a misnomer. The concept 'underclass' denies the unifying element of the working class so central to Marxist analysis, which in turn leaves open the route to the plural working *classes* – segmented social groupings with discrete interests and goals. However, Rogers (1988) has demonstrated that the imputed separate interests or divisiveness inherent in resorting to 'underclass' is not a tenable argument, citing a number of instances of solidarity between full-time and 'underclass' workers, and the underlying potential for class unity. Moreover, when full-time workers struggle successfully, the part-time and the unemployed – including blacks – also benefit; not least because jobs are preserved, as well as improvements in pay and conditions (Cliff 1957). There are a number of instances of 'core' white workers supporting 'underclass' black workers – as in the famous example of the Grunwick dispute of 1977. For Marxists, the unifying element of the working class stems from its relationship to the means of production, namely it does not own or control them: this being true both of the employed and unemployed elements. But unity in struggle, is never considered ineluctable, being rather a function of social conditions and consciousness – including the politics of the protagonists – prevailing at any given point in time. Where these combine in a positive manner, class unity is possible; and this best occurs during periods of unrest and struggle such as in times of riots or strikes.

But emphasis on class does not imply glossing over the import of race; on the contrary, Marxists stress the importance of the racial oppression of black people – and how this is the prime cause of their registering worse on every socio-economic indicator, which in turn explains why so many rioters are black. The classical Marxist Leon Trotsky argued in the 1930s that the social position of blacks meant that they would be at the forefront of many confrontations and rebellions. He argued that blacks in America 'are convoked by the historic development to become a vanguard of the working class' and that they 'in any case will fight better than the white workers' (Trotsky 1989: 62, 30). To understand the impulse to specifically black discontent and unrest of the period under discussion, a brief sketch of blacks in Britain is worthwhile.

The majority of black migrants arrived in Britain after the Second World War. Despite many of them being 'skilled' workers, they found themselves overwhelmingly located in unskilled and semi-skilled jobs. This was during the post-war reconstruction and the start of the long boom, when the British economy suffered from labour shortages. A combination of, at first, right-wing racism and later, the slowing down of the economy, gave impetus to 'concern over immigration' and the passing of immigration controls – inherently racist because they applied only to blacks – so that the presence of blacks began increasingly to be perceived as a 'problem' (Foot 1965; Miles and Phizacklea 1984). This was tantamount to an important denial of the rights of black people in that great barriers were put in their ability to bring members of their families to Britain. Moreover, it accentuated divisions in the working class and provided a potential for blacks to be scapegoated – which the Tory right and, especially, pro-Nazi organizations systematically did after the onset of the first major post-war economic crisis in 1973. An important consequence of this was a deepening in black alienation and feeling of rejection from mainstream society; heightened by the repressive policing of black communities. Another economic crisis ensued in 1979, leading to historically high levels of unemployment and intensifying attacks on the welfare state, both assisted in good measure by the new Conservative government. This disproportionally affected low-skilled workers, hence dispropor-tionally affected black workers. In its wake, present and future prospects for black youth became extremely gloomy, whose unem-ployment rate rose to a multiple of the national average. They, however, were second or third generation migrants, and were not prepared to put up with racial and economic injustice. Instead, there ensued an intensification of the opposition to racism, and the vociferous demands for, and expectation of, equal rights and status – akin to what blacks had done in America in the 1960s. In summary, the system in crisis, in conjunction with rising and systemic police harassment of blacks, provided the dynamic behind black rejection of the *status quo* and the willingness to rebel and riot.

Marxist analysis denies the conservative and liberal/social-democratic view of riots being 'irrational' or 'mindless' acts committed by 'mobs'; as 'aberrations' from the self-correcting harmony and equilibrium of capitalist society. On the contrary, the class nature of society implies continual disequilibria so that conflict ebbs and flows according to prevailing societal conditions. The theory predicts and history provides ample evidence for such persistent disequilibria. From this perspective, therefore, protest against social injustice – a fundamental expression of class struggle – is 'rational' when no other meaningful alternatives to address and rectify grievances are available. Rudé (1964: 6) states the riot is an 'ever-recurring form of popular protest which, on occasion, turns into rebellion or revolution'. Marxist historians have examined riots in both pre- and post-industrial societies, suggesting that they were, in the eighteenth century (prior to the formation of trade unions), a form of 'collective bargaining' (ibid.: 70). In contrast, modern urban riots (in developed countries) can be considered struggles to improve general social conditions and as such constitute a form of class struggle outside the workplace (Harman 1981: 6).

However, unlike the pre-twentieth-century riots, modern riots in parliamentary democracies are a form of popular protest where at least nominal universal political rights do exist. We may therefore assert that, ultimately, they have strong economic roots; encompassing demands not only for social, but economic justice on which the former is predicated. Hence, the denial of adequate material conditions in the sense of a societal/historical norm – with little hope for improvement in the future – provides the impulse for protest which is compounded by an unsympathetic political regime and repressive state apparatus, especially the police, which attempts to impose its authority in the face of opposition; to ensure the restoration of order and control in the event of unrest. However, the class divide becomes accentuated in conflagrations so that the perceived neutrality of the state is exposed as a fallacy which also contemporaneously sees the 'coming together' of different strands of those communities under assault – both black and white – in a show of collective and class solidarity. Where riots are localized, the state can control them with relative ease; but where they become generalized – encompassing broad swathes of the working class – they can escalate into major conflagrations, in which case all the forces of the state are needed for their submission. In this sense riots are minor revolts, and the urgent and crucial task of the state is to prevent their breaking out into, in Rudé's words, rebellion or revolution: in sum, to ensure the safety, above all, of property and the propertied. Moreover, in viewing riots as invariably a class rebellion of the oppressed and exploited – of both employed and unemployed – there is the recognition that benefits which accrue from this struggle are benefits in general for the working class, such as increased resources, including employment and better facilities. None the less, even if the carrot of some material benefits is granted by the state (see next section), alongside the stick of repression, this will not put an end to future unrest and riots as long as the system remains intact. For Marxists, abolition of riots depends on nothing less than the removal of capitalism by working-class revolution and its replacement with a socialist society free from oppression and exploitation.

Though Marx had argued that 'material being determines consciousness', there is none the less a deficiency in the analysis in explaining precisely how this arises, of what processes lead to riotous behaviour. Even if we accept that certain material conditions are necessary for a predisposition towards social conflict, this is not 'sufficient' to explain when and why a certain type of conflict – such as riots – should occur. As Saunders asks (Waddington *et al.* 1989: 178): why do the same system contradictions give rise to 'wild' spontaneous reactions in one area, to organized political movements in another, and to apathetic resignation in a third? Reicher's (1984; 1996) 'social identity model' and Waddington *et al.*'s (1989) 'flashpoints' model help provide the answers and are also useful in making the link between being, consciousness and action. The importance of 'interaction' between groups is of crucial importance here. Waddington *et al.* argue that disorder stems from the occurrence of a 'flashpoint' which they deem to be a 'dramatic break in a pattern of "interaction" which might itself help to explain why and where disorder broke out' (1989: 21). Reicher emphasizes social categories and intergroup dynamics between the 'in-group' (demonstrators, rioters) and the 'out-group' (invariably, the police) arguing that it is the pattern of action and reaction that leads to violence (1996: 124). Moreover, 'the spread of conflict coincides in the self-categorisation of crowd members' – how a fragmented crowd becomes largely homogenous (Reicher 1996: 129, 130). If we equate social category with class, this, in Marxist terminology, becomes especially useful in explicating the movement from 'class in itself' to 'class for itself' in moments of struggle.

The impact of riots

Riots have occurred throughout the period under discussion in this chapter. The serious and widespread nature of the 1981 riots provoked the Conservative government to take ameliorative measures, recognizing that condemnation alone would not suffice to diffuse the situation. In this, the government followed the American government when it set up the Kerner Commission in 1968, though the nature of the British government's measures was much less in comparison. The Home Secretary, William Whitelaw, authorized an urgent inquiry led by Lord Scarman to look into the disorders in Brixton and make recommendations. Scarman was well-known for his liberal sympathies, so the government hoped his appointment would appease critics of any bias: this proved largely to be the case within Parliament, though there were critics outside, including black groupings and commentators. Scarman completed the Report in November 1981, concluding that:

> the social conditions in Brixton ... do not provide an excuse for disorder ... all those who in the course of the disorders in Brixton and elsewhere engaged in violence against the police were guilty of grave criminal offences.
>
> (Scarman 1981: 2.31)

Thus, a significant proportion of the Report deals with policing matters and law reform. And he makes it clear that the spark which ignited the riots in Brixton came from 'a spontaneous act of defiant aggression by young men who felt themselves hunted by a hostile police force' (ibid.: 3.25). None the less, he did recognize that the lives of ethnic minority groups:

> are led largely in the poorer and more deprived areas of our great cities. Unemployment and poor housing bear on them very heavily and the educational system has not adjusted itself satisfactorily to their needs. Their difficulties are intensified by the sense they have of a concealed discrimination against them, particularly in relation to job opportunities and housing. ... Taken together they

provide a set of social 'conditions' which create a predisposition towards violent protest.

(Scarman 1981: 2.35, 2.38)

Following from this, Scarman recommends that 'positive action' needs to be undertaken to alleviate problems of housing, education and employment, together with the tackling of racial discrimination that underpins these (1981: Part VI, especially 6.10–6.37). The measures offered were, however, severely limited in scope or, as Lea and Young put it, just 'timid' (1982: 20). One – perhaps the main – reason for this was that Scarman did not 'consider it appropriate to make recommendations about the scale of resources which should be devoted to either inner city or ethnic minority needs. It is for Government and Parliament in the final analysis to judge the relative priority they should be given' (1981: 6.33). But he did later caution that 'if the recommendations in his report were not broadly followed, there could be serious trouble in some inner city areas' (*Financial Times*, 27 February 1982).

The Scarman Report, as Taylor (1984: 30) has commented, embodies different theoretical explanations of 'collective violence' (that is, of riots). But with regard to the recommendations, it is a combination of liberal/social-democratic and conservative interpretations. Liberal/social-democratic in the sense of favouring reform of institutions and the channelling of additional resources towards deprived groups; and conservative in the sense of advocating new tactics and equipment for the police to make them more effective in tackling future riots. This approach resulted in all the major political parties and mainstream commentators broadly being in favour of the Report (the Report was welcomed by both the Home Secretary William Whitelaw and the Shadow Home Secretary Roy Hattersley; the Metropolitan Police Commissioner, Sir David McNee, described the Report as fair and thorough; while the media reaction was generally very positive (Kettle and Hodges 1982: 208)). However, because of Scarman's refusal to countenance fundamental problems of the polity – of giving air to the 'radical' views – the Report was bound to fall far short of acceptance by those not adhering to the liberal/social-democratic/conservative consensus – almost exclusively of those on the left – including black community representatives and groups (for example, the Brixton Defence Committee called for a boycotting of the Scarman Inquiry from the outset, fearing its limited nature and attempts at 'whitewashing' the core problems (*Financial Times*, 16 April 1981)). But Scarman's own warning of future trouble, if his recommendations were not implemented, was manifestly justified as widespread riots erupted again in 1985. Prashar (1987) castigated the government for its failure to take the 'positive action' for racial minorities as advocated by Scarman. Benyon and Solomos (1987: 194) have observed that there was little sign of the commitment to remove the roots of urban unrest, that is, to tackle the adverse socio-economic and political conditions which were still so prevalent in the major cities. Indeed, not only were Scarman's social measures not implemented, there were no further governmental inquiries established, nor promises made of injections of significant investments and resources for inner cities. Thus, after the riots in Handsworth in 1985, the Home Secretary Douglas Hurd opted for a police inquiry which, unsurprisingly, focused on issues related to drugs, crime and general lawlessness of the area (Dear 1985).

The Conservative government, boosted by a huge parliamentary majority in the 1983 election, had reverted to an orthodox conservative, 'condemnatory' stance – to the exclusion of social factors. Its stress on crime as a mainspring of the riots began to dominate (Solomos 1986: 24). Moreover, since it was elected on a tax-cutting promise, there was little likelihood of systematic injections of government funding for the inner cities. The market was to be the chief allocator of resources – and the government assiduously argued that its role would be to deregulate markets and reduce company taxes in conjunction with strict control of inflation for macro-economic stability. These, it believed, were the key incentives for inducing private investment throughout the economy – including inner cities. Workers would, therefore, need to acquire relevant skills and accept wages that the market determined – of not pricing themselves out of jobs (Robins 1985).

However, this market-centred policy for the inner cities proved far from successful: on the contrary, their overall condition continued to worsen. This, indeed, was the conclusion of a major report conducted by the Department of Environment's Inner Cities Research Programme whose aim it was to evaluate the overall impact of central government urban policy in England during the 1980s and early 1990s. Their sample was 123 English local authorities – but the study focused on the 57 Urban Priority Areas (that is, the most deprived) that were the target of the government's Action for Cities Package. Though the results of the research show a 'mixed picture', the crucial conclusion is clear: 'indications of deteriorating conditions in the UPAs over the period as a whole' (Department of Environment 1994: vii). None the less, the immediate aftermath of riots can bring some material benefits. As Power and Tunstall show in their study, riot-torn areas, rather than being 'punished' by government for the breakdown of order, did win additional support, though they go on to acknowledge that this had a limited impact because it 'did not tackle the underlying social and economic problems, and ... did little to change the status or attitude of the excluded and troublesome young men' (1997: 23–4).

But in some senses, the impact of riots can be thought of as providing other, less material, benefits. One benefit in Britain was that the Conservatives never played the 'race card' as blatantly as they had done during the 1960s and 1970s, or as Margaret Thatcher had done in her 'alien culture' comment; this mainly became the preserve of the far-right and the conservative press. There became established a general acceptance of the black British presence in mainstream political circles. Another benefit is that riots can unify blacks and whites (provided they are not 'race riots' where, as is invariably the case, whites assault black people): as already noted, in mixed areas, multiracial riots have been the norm for the period under discussion. This has the benefit of reducing racial divisions, hence of scapegoating, so that not only blacks, but whites also potentially benefit from resistance to divisive policies. At the same time, there can be a reduction in police harassment, as the government exhorts – at least in the immediate aftermath of riots – the police to be more 'sensitive', fearful of another bout of riots being triggered through police aggression (though this needs to be offset against the broader picture of an increasingly well-armed and militarized police force that became a hallmark of Conservative policing methods – to coincide with its stress on law and order issues). And the experience of struggling against injustice and repression can lead to a positive 'transformation in consciousness' (Harman 1981: 40) where, for example, white racism is challenged, and there is the potential for less friction between the various black communities. This can have long-term consequences, especially the realization of class interests irrespective of race or creed – a sense of the class acting for itself.

However, the benefits flowing from this form of class struggle should not be exaggerated. Harman (1981: 37) has provided the striking metaphor that 'riots rise up like rockets but drop like a stick' – that is, they end rapidly invariably within days. The analogy suggests that benefits that are reaped in the aftermath of riots are less specific and often short-lived.

Conclusion

From our survey of the major theories of riots, we rejected conservative explanations as providing a satisfactory account, stemming from their inadequate consideration of socio-economic and political factors. Liberal/social-democratic and black nationalist theories, though starting from different perspectives, do take these factors as being key to an understanding of riots and civil unrest, and both advocate reform of institutions, though in the latter case there is always the recognition that this may not be satisfactory. Though race and community are accorded dominance the black nationalist view nonetheless acknowledges the importance of class, but its analysis is weakened by invoking the inadequate concept of the 'black underclass'. The Marxian perspective's primacy on class analysis sets it apart from other explanations, this gives it greater consistency and insight. The recognition that a section of the working class – especially the unorganized and the unemployed, often from minority ethnic communities – might at certain junctures resort to riots where 'normal' channels and institutions fail, is a more convincing explanation than that provided by the other theories which do not locate the specificities of the riot as opposed to other forms of protest. The experience of British riots of the 1980s and 1990s with its interracial mix adds support to this view by showing the forging of unity between blacks and whites. This phenomenon was also evident in America following the major Los Angeles' riot in 1992 that triggered a spate of riots throughout America, for these too were multiracial – showing the emergence of unity between groups which previously had had a history of profound hostility towards each other (Davis 1992). What this suggests is that when faced with deep grievances, revolt can generalize to different sections of communities, that ordinarily might view one another as hostile competitors. With respect to riots, we might conclude that the struggle against injustice gives impetus to unity and helps explain the 'contagion effect' as they spread from district to district and city to city, in the process drawing in different groups. None the less, existing Marxist theory has paid less attention to precisely how riots occur, and I have argued that Waddington *et al.*'s (1989) and Reicher's (1984; 1996) theories emphasizing group interaction provide a helpful schema for overcoming this lacuna.

We can conclude by asserting that against the background of historically high levels of unemployment, sluggish economic growth punctuated by severe recessions, and the persistence of endemic racism, not only in Britain but in all the advanced economies, the 'reservoir of grievances' among the oppressed and exploited is likely to remain deep – in turn providing the material basis for future riots and revolts.

Notes

1   I would like to offer my thanks to Colin Barker, Jenny Taylor and Gerry Mooney for their many helpful suggestions.
2   It must be stressed at the outset, however, that though this analysis is largely adhered to by those supporting Liberal Democratic and Labour parties in Britain, it may also include some from those supporting the Conservatives – and conversely, at times – those who ostensibly espouse this view can also adopt conservative 'law and order' explanations, as is often the case with leading politicians in the immediate aftermath of riots (as did for example Roy Hattersley and Jeff Rooker following the Totten-ham riots in 1985 (Benyon and Solomos 1987: 11)).
3   In the discussion which follows I engage with the term 'underclass' as used by Sivanandan (1981/2), to refer to the racially 'excluded', revolutionary black youth of the inner cities. More recently, of course, the term 'underclass' has been associated with sociologists like Charles Murray and right-wing politicians who use it to refer to, in the words of Bagguley and Mann (1992), 'the idle, thieving, bastards', the 'welfare dependent' who populate inner-city housing estates. Sivanandan's usage, it should be made clear, is quite distinct from such reactionary conceptualizations of the term.

11 'No poll tax here!'

The Tories, social policy and the great poll tax rebellion 1987–1991

Michael Lavalette and Gerry Mooney

> The Poll Tax is Thatcher's Flagship as was the Titanic the British Naval Flagship. They said the flagship was unsinkable as they say that Thatcher is unbeatable. But the Titanic was sunk by an ice-berg and so will the poll tax be sunk by an ice-berg. A human ice-berg of mass non-payment. ... Raise your sights, join our campaign. The time to fight back is now!
>
> (Strathclyde Anti-Poll Tax Federation 1989: 41–2)

Introduction

There is an increasingly powerful myth which suggests that the 1980s was the decade of yuppies, enrichment and the victory of Thatcherite ideals. Yet these claims hide the fact that the decade was one of growing inequality and was punctured by significant social conflict. In January 1980, the decade opened with a steel strike. This was followed by massive demonstrations against unemployment, urban riots and a number of 'days of action' called by the Trades Union Congress (TUC), under the moderate leadership of Len Murray. In 1982 and 1983 there were a series of rolling regional general strikes in support of hospital workers and against attempts to privatize parts of the National Health Service (NHS). Indeed, in September 1982 the *Financial Times* estimated that 2 million workers had come out on strike on the 22 September in support of health workers. As the decade continued there were significant strikes in the newspaper and railway industries, on the docks and, of course, in the mines where the *Financial Times* described the level of support for the strikers as 'the biggest and most continuous civilian mobilisation to confront the government since the Second World War' (quoted in Jones and Novak 1985: 99). Teachers and local government workers struck against privatization, changes to working conditions, over pay levels and against the imposition (in the case of teachers) of the National Curriculum and the testing of pupils via Standard Attainment Tests (SATs). The decade ended with a rebellion against the imposition of a local 'community charge' or poll tax, which, at its height, involved 17 million adults refusing to pay a legal tax. It is certainly true that many of these conflicts ended in defeat for organized workers, but it is not the case that the Thatcher-led Conservative governments were easily able to roll over the working-class movement.

Yet despite much of this, in the mid-1980s there developed a powerful set of arguments, primarily by writers associated with the journal *Marxism Today*, which suggested that 'Thatcherism', embodying a new 'hegemonic project', had successfully marginalized opposition and been instrumental in establishing 'New Times' (Hall and Jacques 1989). These ideas suggested that Thatcherism had successfully broken the post-war consensus developed around a commitment to the Keynes-Beveridgean welfare state and had established new shared values around 'authoritarian populism', individualism and the creation of a 'share-owning, property-owning' democracy.

The evidence for such claims was always (at best) contradictory. From 1983 onwards, repeated British Social Attitude Survey Reports suggested that substantial sections of the population remained deeply committed to collective provision of welfare. The surveys show continuing commitment to the NHS and an adequately funded education system; to tackling the problem of unemployment rather than scapegoating the unemployed; and to support for state pensions and disability benefits rather than various 'welfare to work' schemes (Sullivan 1996).

The various movements mentioned above also demonstrate that there was always a substantial and active minority who rejected the 'Thatcher agenda'; nor is it the case that these movements always ended in defeat or that the Thatcher governments were invincible. During the miners' strike there were several points where victory over the government was a very real possibility (Callinicos and Simons 1985), the devastation of the dock industry can at least partially be blamed on union prevarication (Lavalette and Kennedy 1996), and the strikes and actions of activists within the health and education services limited, to some degree, the extent to which the Tories' privatization agenda was introduced and implemented.

The poll tax rebellion provides further evidence of the failure of Thatcherism to obtain hegemony. The poll tax became Thatcher's flagship. It reflected a number of core Tory values around notions of individualism, control of local government spending, increasing inequality and transferring the tax burden on to the working class. The confrontations it engendered, the mass campaign of non-payment, the conflicts at town halls across the country, the massive demonstrations and the 'Battle of Trafalgar', led to the tax being removed and was the central element that led the Tories to ditch Margaret Thatcher from her prime ministerial position.

Yet at the time, the anti-poll tax movement was interpreted by some academics as a 'new' non-class-based social movement, or alternatively, as the revolt of 'middle England' (despite the fact that the campaign started in Scotland) against an unjust tax (for many of these themes, see Hoggett and Burns 1991; Burns 1992; Baggley 1996). This is a position we reject. In this chapter we trace the creation of the tax and look at the form and composition of the anti-tax movement. We argue that the poll tax needs to be set in an appropriate context as a piece of anti-working class legislation and that class is central to any understanding of its unequal consequences for prospective payers and to the campaign against its imposition: the anti-poll tax movement was an overwhelmingly working-class mobilization against a central piece of government taxation policy. We start by outlining the context within which the tax developed in order to argue that it represented a key piece of Tory legislation structured around central social policy goals inherent in their project.

The Tories and social policy: goals, perspectives and 'real politick'

When the Conservative Party was elected in May 1979 it was against a backdrop of Labour cuts in welfare, with schools, hospitals and local authorities all finding their budgets squeezed by Dennis Healey's monetarist policies. Labour's compulsory incomes policies saw workers' living standards decline in real terms. In the winter of 1978/79, there was a rebellion of the low paid against Labour's austerity measures known as the 'Winter of Discontent' (see Cliff and Gluckstein 1988).

For a substantial section of both the Tory Party and the dominant class in Britain, the new government had to address a number of serious economic and political problems if the British economy's apparent terminal decline was to be reversed: low rates of both profitability and productivity; a recent history of stagflation; a substantial sector of the economy dominated by unprofitable, nationalized industries; a powerful trade union movement and a working class who expected welfare to expand and their wages to increase, year on year. Sir John Methven, Director-General of the Confederation of British Industry, said in November 1979: 'Britain on the eve of the 1980's ... [is] poised between remorseless decline and real success, between disintegration and moral recovery' (quoted in Harman 1985: 73). And arch-Thatcherite Keith Joseph is quoted as saying of the pre-1979 era: 'We were over-governed, over-taxed, over-borrowed, over-manned, under-defended, under-policed and rather badly educated' (quoted in Timmins 1996: 371).

In the first four months of 1979, *The Economist* magazine made repeated calls for a wage freeze, denationalization policies, reductions in social spending and a concerted attempt to control union power. For example, on 13 January 1979, the magazine's editorial made the following argument:

> A sensible way to break the wage inflation spiral would be a six month wage freeze. ... [further] There is a growing consensus between Mr Callaghan and Mrs Thatcher that the reduction of union bargaining power is at the heart of any government's anti-inflation policy.
>
> (*The Economist*, 13 January 1979: 17–18)

While the first Tory White Paper of 1979 stated that 'Public expenditure is at the heart of Britain's present economic difficulties' (quoted in Timmins 1996: 371). Thus, part of the Tory agenda was to reassert the profitability of British capitalism by trying to restrain working-class wages and reduce public social spending: to solve the economic crisis by increasing the exploitation of working-class families and curtailing the social wage.

Tory economic policy was structured around 'monetarism' and 'supply side economics'. In broad terms, the monetarist part involved an attempt to control the money supply to reduce inflation and control the cyclical movement of the economy, putting financial constraints on managers to force them to shed labour and reduce wage costs. The second element entailed reducing government intervention in the economy as much as possible, cutting taxation and attacking 'monopoly players' (especially the trade unions who, they claimed, introduced disequilibrium into the labour market), all of which would increase the 'supply side' incentives to entrepreneurs, and would in turn create economic boom conditions and balance government budgets.

The Tories' perspectives on social policy were structured ideologically around four interrelated concerns. First, to increase inequality. The pursuit of equality and welfare expansion, they suggested, had created a culture of welfare dependency which had undermined the entrepreneurial spirit in Britain and, both directly and indirectly, had undermined economic performance. Second, to control local government. They suggested that local government had expanded, was inefficient and was run by local, 'amateur' politicians, often pursuing extreme political agendas. Education and social work services, for example, had come under the influence of the so-called 'loony left', promoting minority cultures, life-styles and 'anti-British' or 'non-traditional' values. Third, state welfare bureaucracies, cocooned from market imperatives, were inefficient and ineffective and had to be 'reformed' to reflect market imperatives. They suggested that welfare expansion had led to the growth of unaccountable bureaucracies pursuing their own interests and defining the needs of others (patients, clients and users). What was needed was a 'consumer' and 'customer' orientation where an individual's wants would be met by market methods of provision. Finally, 'socialism' was to be eradicated. The term 'socialism' was used loosely to refer to a range of political opponents and forms of organization which the Thatcherites thought expressed a 'collectivist ethos': trade unions, nationalized industries, all forms of collective welfare provision, the Keynesian-Beveridgean settlement, the Labour Party, 'old style' local government. The social-democratic consensus had to be smashed and replaced by a shared commitment to a 'home owning, share owning democracy' built around the values of individualism.

As Timmins makes clear, Thatcher shared these social policy goals from the earliest days of her first government. From various interviews he conducted with Cabinet and Junior Ministers we find that:

'She had a sense that it cost a lot [the welfare state] ... she did have a feeling that individual initiative and drive for self-improvement could be undermined by too extensive a welfare state; that it could rot people's moral fibre' [David Willetts]. ... 'She did have this feeling about the insurance principle, that people who could afford to should insure themselves' [Norman Fowler]. ... 'She *hated* the Department of Education' ... [and favoured the idea of school vouchers] [Stuart Sexton]. ... 'She thought it was disgraceful that people who could afford it relied on the taxpayer to provide their health' [Kenneth Clarke].

(Quoted in Timmins 1996: 372–4)

Both the economic and social policy objectives were interconnected and overlapped. But while these perspectives shaped the *goals* of Tory economic and social policy, they were tempered in practice as a consequence of the difficulties (or perceived difficulties) and opposition engendered by the political process. This was especially so with regard to their social policy agenda. Thus one of the notable features of the first two Tory governments was its failure (in their terms) to cut social spending significantly. In part this was a consequence of the depth of the Labour cuts in the 1976–1979 period (hence there was little room for 'easy' cuts in services with many reductions in spending and provision provoking opposition, either nationally or locally). It also reflected spiralling unemployment and poverty and the consequent rise in social security spending. But it was also a result of Thatcher's *caution* – her belief that the welfare state was immensely popular and that marketization could prove politically costly, or provoke a generalized defence from the organized working-class movement, points emphasized by Willetts, Fowler, Sexton and Clarke in their interviews with Timmins (1996).

Thus the priority became tackling the unions, denationalization policies, reducing taxation, reducing payments to 'lame duck' industries and reducing labour costs (primarily via 'market methods', that is the threat of unemployment). As one of Thatcher's key supporters notes:

> She was adamant that she would not start down this sort of road at the beginning [i.e. privatizing the welfare state]. There was enough to do sorting out industry, the economy, taxation and the trade unions. 'The supply side must come first' she said.
>
> (Nicholas Ridley, quoted in Timmins 1996: 372)

Even on the question of reducing workers' wages the Conservative government's successes were limited in the early years of power. Indeed, in summer 1982 *The Economist* highlighted this failing and suggested that the government needed to cut wages by an average of 20 per cent to restore profitability levels for British capital. It was the poor working class, those in marginal jobs, part-time work or the increasing numbers facing periods of unemployment in the early 1980s, who saw their standard of living fall dramatically. As Harman argued in 1985, Thatcher faced a paradox:

> one reason she had been able to win the general election of 1983 was because she could boast to many workers that they were as

well off as they had ever been; yet that was the opposite of the goals she had set for British capitalism.

(Harman 1985: 81–2)

We are not arguing that the Tory governments of 1979–1987 did not alter the shape of British politics, did not inflict significant defeats on the British working-class movement and did not increase inequality, unemployment and poverty – clearly they did all of these things. But some of the changes have certainly been exaggerated and in the area of social policy, with the exception of housing, Johnson felt able to state that after two Tory administrations: 'the welfare state has not yet been dismantled. The major services, much changed and with inadequate resources, are still in place' (1990: 225).

1987: social policy 'watershed'?

Nevertheless, the social policy goals remained and in the run up to the election in 1987 the Tories turned their sights more fully to welfare provision. Sullivan (1996) notes that four key social policy areas (the poll tax, further housing reform, school 'opt-out' and NHS reform) all figured centrally in the 1987 Tory Manifesto as social welfare reform moved to centre stage.

In a number of reviews of Tory social policy changes, 1987 is identified as a 'watershed' year (Le Grand 1990; Deakin 1994; Ellison and Pierson 1998). Deakin suggests that:

The new policy initiatives outlined in the 1987 manifesto and their successors represented a decision to bring the solvent of market conditions to bear on the problems of the welfare system.

(Deakin 1994: 153)

But while social policy commentators have identified the 1987 manifesto as the turning point for social welfare there has been less attention given to explaining *why* the Tories waited until 1987/88 before launching their 'welfare offensive'. Deakin suggests it was the consequence of their continuing electoral success and the size of their parliamentary majority (1994: 156). While at least recognizing that there is an important issue to be addressed, Deakin's analysis is curtailed by his inability to look beyond parliamentary politics and procedures (indeed, the Manifesto commitments obviously came before the size of their majority was realized). For others, the first two terms of Tory government had been addressed to solving Britain's economic problems; by 1987 these were complete and the government could turn to social welfare. But this analysis exaggerates the 'economic successes' of the Tory years and, in reality, does no more than repeat Tory propaganda about the 'economic miracle' (see Wilson 1992).

It is our contention that the developments of 1987 can only be fully comprehended within the context of political opposition and the ebb and flow of class conflict as they manifested themselves in the mid-1980s. There were two interrelated elements to this process, which, for simplicity, we can conceptualize as a 'political' opposition around the left of the Labour Party and an 'industrial' opposition, referring to the level and intensity of industrial conflict.[1]

As Barker and Dale (1999) note, by the end of the 1970s the wave of struggle and protest which had erupted in the late 1960s was receding: there was a marked 'downturn' in the level and intensity of the class struggle. Faced with this situation activists had to reconsider their strategies for achieving social improvement. For many of those in the women's, black, gay and trade union movement, it meant some form of accommodation with the Labour Party. After the victory of Margaret Thatcher in the 1979 election, there was a remarkable growth in the size and influence of the left within the Labour Party. This was expressed most clearly in the movement around Tony Benn to win the deputy leadership and to introduce democratic control and accountability within the Party. It also led to the growth of a brand of 'local municipal socialism' (primarily in a number of city authorities in England), where left-wing local councils used the rates to raise money to defend and promote a range of 'progressive' causes (Boddy and Fudge 1984). For example, the Greater London Council (GLC) under Ken Livingstone promoted subsidized transport (until prohibited from doing so by national government), had a distinct 'Industrial and Financial Strategy' for London's regeneration and promoted a range of equal opportunities policies (GLC, 1985). David Blunkett in Sheffield led a council that followed a similar strategy, while in Liverpool, the Militant Tendency were able to gain control of the council and redirect some welfare spending towards, for example, a limited house building programme. Without exaggerating the resistance of these councils to national government (which was often very short lived), they were increasingly portrayed as a source of opposition to the Tories' economic goal of reducing government spending, by dint of the councils' monetary raising powers and budget plans, and to the government's ideological pursuit of privatization, marketization and individualism. The Tories responded by 'rate-capping', reducing local government grants and even, in the case of the GLC, by abolition.

But the left-wing councils were also under attack from the leadership of the Labour Party. For Labour Party 'modernizers', left-wing councils were undermining Labour's credibility as a 'party of government': all opposition from Labour had to be 'legitimate', it had to stick by the normal rules of parliamentary democracy. The consequence was that the Labour leadership increasingly distanced themselves from strikes (most notably the miners' strike of 1984/85), demonstrations and local government 'extremism'. For Labour leader Neil Kinnock it was better for Labour councils to carry out cuts and government policy rather than oppose them which could antagonize the Tories and lead to increasing centralization.

With hindsight, we can see that the Labour leadership's strategy did nothing to stop the diminution of local government power. But the key point to note is that the municipal left were under attack from both the Tories and the Labour leadership. The central period in the struggle of the left councils was the spring and summer of 1984/85, when a number of councils refused to set a legal rate in a direct challenge to the government. The government was under intense pressure due to the miners' strike and the possibilities of a united opposition were substantial. But one by one the councils capitulated to pressure from the national Labour leadership, or succumbed to short-term amelioratives from the Tories. By 1986 Liverpool council was isolated, vulnerable and eventually defeated. The influence of the Labour left was declining sharply and the age of New Labour was dawning.

The industrial confrontations were more visible and dramatic than those taking place in the council chambers. In the early Thatcher years confrontations between trade unions, employers and government were fairly common, fairly bloody and generally marked by trade union defeat. The 'Ridley Plan', developed by sections of the Tory Party while in opposition, had been clear about any future government's strategy to deal with trade union power. Weaker unions were to be dealt with first, generalized conflicts with the union movement were to be avoided and, if necessary, concessions were to be made to more powerful sections of the unionized workforce until the government was ready to enter into conflict with them. Anti-union legislation would be introduced (again, slowly at first) in an attempt to curtail acts of solidarity and force trade union leaders to police their members. Further, mass unemployment, it was hoped, would discipline workers and reduce their scope for solidarity action.

In the early 1980s the successes of this strategy had weakened the union movement but they had not undermined trade union conscious-ness among substantial layers of workers. The steel strike, which lasted for fourteen weeks, was far more militant than the government had expected; in 1981 the government was forced to back down to striking South Welsh miners and the skirmishes on the railways, in the health service, civil service and education proved more popular than the government anticipated. In this atmosphere there were clear divisions within the ruling class over the appropriate strategy to follow. These included divisions between:

> the 'Thatcherites and the 'wets' ... [between] those industrialists who wanted state intervention and those who didn't, between financiers who wanted to free themselves from what they saw as a national base in irreversible decline and those who did not, be-tween those who prioritised collaboration with the US and those who thought the only future lay in the creation of a European ruling class ... between those who saw the greatest danger as being the 'disintegration of the national fabric' into bitter class struggle, and those who believed their class would win such struggles.
>
> (Harman 1985: 80)

In this climate, while individual unions had been isolated and defeated, the government still felt vulnerable to a general working-class assault. Cuts and privatization in welfare provision represented an attack on the entire working class and their social wage and contained the *possibility* of provoking a generalized response. This was clearly one important factor preventing such an attack.

What changed at the end of the second Tory government was its confidence in its ability to resist a collective response to welfare reforms and this was a direct consequence of the aftermath of the miners' dispute of 1984/85. The miners' dispute was immensely important for both sides in the class struggle. As German notes, in the aftermath of the strike 'there followed a series of confrontations in which the ruling class went in for the kill' (1990: 21). For the working-class movement, the defeat of the miners was a dreadful blow. The miners were seen as the most important, powerful and militant section of the working class, if they could not defeat the Tories, then, it seemed, no one could. The effect the defeat had on the trade union movement was to strengthen the hand of those who argued for accommodation with the government and employers on their terms, it sapped the confidence of many trade union activists, within the

Labour Party it strengthened the hand of 'new realist' modernizers around Neil Kinnock and seemed to push socialism off the agenda. Victory for the government meant the removal of the single most important union obstacle to its economic and political agenda. And with victory came confidence – the trade union/militant socialist opposition had been defeated, the balance of class forces had shifted decisively in favour of capital and the government. It was now possible to push through radical changes to Britain's social fabric, to push out the last vestiges of the social-democratic consensus and assert the superiority of the values of individualism.

Thus the Thatcherite social policy perspectives and goals came to the fore in the aftermath of their victory over the miners and in the run up to the election in 1987. It was in this context that Thatcher's third-term flagship, the poll tax, was formulated and advanced as a means of reshaping local government, controlling its expenditure and altering the form of local welfare provision. It is to the origins and germination of the poll tax that we now turn.

The origins of the 'community charge'

According to both McConnell (1989) and Midwinter and Monaghan (1993) the poll tax developed essentially as a response to the problem of the 1985 rate revaluation in Scotland, in a context of dwindling Tory Party support and representation. In the post-war era the Tories had declined from the largest party in Scotland to a minority party struggling to maintain a presence among elected Scottish MPs. The 'rates rebellion' was mediated through the Scottish Conservative Party. High rates were viewed as disproportionately affecting traditional Tory supporters while letting profligate Labour councils redirect resources towards services for the poor.

There is no doubt that the continuing decline in Tory fortunes led the Party in Scotland to consider alternatives to the rates as a form of local government finance. It is also useful to remember, in the face of some nationalist arguments which suggest that the poll tax was an attack by English Tories on all Scots, that the initial demands for change came from sections of the Scottish middle and upper classes, who complained that they were paying too much to subsidize the range of local welfare services. Further, abolition of the rates had been the Tory Party's policy position in both the 1974 and 1979 election manifestos. But this fails to answer the question why it was the poll tax, rather than local taxation, for example, that became the government's preferred option. The perceived problems of rate revaluation in Scotland and the demands of the Scottish petite bourgeoisie may have hastened its implementation and may explain why it was introduced in Scotland first, but it is far from being the full story.

Butler *et al.* (1994) suggest that the tax emerged almost accidentally from various government committees. It was an ill-conceived idea. To quote Robert Harris in *The Sunday Times*, it was 'a gaffe, bungle, goof, fluff, fiasco, boner, clanger, howler and flop ... a cock up' (24 February 1991). Butler *et al.* trace the process of the 'emergence' of the tax from a meeting held on 31 March 1985 at Chequers, attended by almost half the Cabinet, where Margaret Thatcher claimed the tax 'was born', to John Major's 1992 election victory, where, they claim, he 'won electoral credit for being the man who got rid of the poll tax' (Butler *et al.* 1994: 301).

They make the suggestion that rate revaluation, north and south of the border, gave impetus to the demand for rate reform by, in particular, George Younger and William Whitelaw. Coincidentally, a review team under the leadership of William Waldegrave suggested a poll tax as a viable means of financing and restructuring local government. The two elements came together and led to a hasty decision to opt for the poll tax. Any doubts about the political viability of the tax were dispelled because of the actions of the socialist municipal councils and their refusal to set a rate in early 1985. The consequence was that:

> The poll tax was elevated from 'bold idea' to 'government policy', in the space of barely three months, because of the enthusiastic backing of the Prime Minister and key colleagues.
>
> (Butler *et al.* 1994: 287)

It is certainly useful to recognize that government policy is not always fully thought out, rational or able to comprehend the range and variety of possible consequences it engenders. But the emphasis on the 'cock-up' theory again fails to locate the development in its context: the Tories' increasing confidence and belief that this was the 'moment' to pursue their social policy agenda. While the rates could have been replaced by any of a range of local taxes, the poll tax most clearly expressed their ideological commitment to redistribute tax, increase inequality and curtail local government spending, thereby controlling left-wing councils.

The poll tax was a clear piece of class legislation. By treating all adults over the age of 18 years as equals it attempted to reinforce the vast social and economic inequalities of wealth and power in society. The effect was to increase further the burden of paying for local welfare services on to the working class and to undermine any notion that tax should be related to income, wealth and ability to pay. To illustrate, the *Guardian* newspaper noted that:

> The Duke of Westminster, who used to pay £10,255 in rates on his estate has just learned his new poll tax: £417. His house-keeper and resident chauffeur face precisely the same bill.
>
> (Quoted in Burns 1992: 10)

In an earlier article on the first year of the poll tax (Lavalette and Mooney 1989) we produced the following table to emphasize the level of change the poll tax introduced.

Table 11.1 The effects of the poll tax on a couple paying average domestic rate bill (selected Scottish districts)

District	Poll tax, two people 1989–1990 (£ per year)	Average domestic rate bill 1988–89 (£ per year)	% increase
Glasgow	612	506	20
Edinburgh	784	603	30
Dundee	684	486	34
Aberdeen	608	432	41
Dunfermline	586	465	26
Falkirk	518	427	21
Lochaber	474	359	32
Berwickshire	472	355	33
Wigtown	493	355	39
Orkney	296	194	52

These increases were based on two people paying the tax, but all people over the age of 18 years were liable to pay – even those on income support had to pay at least 20 per cent. Thus many working-class families faced steeper bills than these figures indicate. Further, the first bills were lower than they would be in preceding years due to government subsidy to aid the transition to the new tax. The situation was clear, the poll tax represented an immense extra burden on working-class families, a burden which many simply could not carry.

In an attempt to stop the poll tax being 'too excessive', the government introduced poll tax capping, the direct effect of which was to force local governments to reduce their social spending. As Burns notes: 'It was not "coincidental" that all the councils capped in the first year were Labour controlled' (1992: 12). In the large towns and cities, the effect of capping was to squeeze services for the very poorest communities. Working-class communities were now expected to pay more tax for a deteriorating service.

Thus, in practice, the poll tax was adopted by the Tories because it suited their wider political agenda and was implemented at a point when they were confident in their ability to resist any opposition the tax might generate. Any such hopes, however, were to be short lived.

The anti-poll tax campaigns: goals, strategies and tactics

Many histories of collective struggles portray the episode(s) in an almost teleological fashion: the great victory, or the 'heroic' defeat, was inevitable from the start, all that is required is to describe the path followed by the actors involved. The problem with such approaches, however, is that they underplay the dynamism of collective action, the intense political debate that it engenders and the competing ideologies and strategies that are promoted by all those involved (both insurgents and opponents) (for an expansion on these themes, see Barker *et al.* forthcoming, b). In the movement against the poll tax we can identify five campaigns against the tax. Ostensibly each had the same goal: abolition. But the ideologies shaping the campaigns and the strategies and tactics followed were radically different in each case. The five campaigns were: one that tied in with the Labour election campaign of June 1987; the 'Stop It' campaign run by the Labour Party in Scotland and the Scottish Trades Union Council (STUC); the Scottish National Party's 'Can Pay, Won't Pay' campaign; 'Committees of 100'; and the mass campaign of non-payment organized by the Anti-Poll Tax Unions (APTUs). These campaigns competed with each other to establish hegemony within the anti-tax campaign in Scotland, as the tax was introduced in Scotland a year before England and Wales. By the time the movement had spread to England and Wales, the APTUs had established hegemony over the anti-poll tax campaign and represented a truly mass social movement.

The Labour Party and the 1987 election

The legislation introducing the poll tax to Scotland was one of the last measures of the second Thatcher government. Although the legislation applied only to Scotland, it was clear that if the Tories were re-elected then England and Wales would follow suit. In these circumstances one might have expected the poll tax to feature prominently in Labour's election campaign in June 1987. Surprisingly, it was rarely mentioned. As some Labour members noted after the election:

> In England the Poll Tax was barely mentioned. In Scotland it was a Bogey Man with which to ensure a good Labour turn-out ... the policy was simple – Vote Labour to Stop the Poll Tax.
>
> (Labour Briefing Scotland 1988: 31)

No consideration was given as to what to do if the Tories won the election as such talk was deemed defeatist. Indeed, at the time, there was much discussion of the 'doomsday scenario': the idea that, if the Tories won the election and Scotland voted Labour 'normal' bourgeois politics would collapse as Scotland would be ungovernable to a third Tory government with no mandate.

At the election Scotland was indeed presented with the 'doomsday scenario'. Labour won an unprecedented fifty seats and the MPs took the self-proclaimed title the 'Fighting 50'. In the euphoria of their success in Scotland many leading Labour MPs felt confident that the Tories would have to retreat. George Foulkes, for example, a traditional right-of-centre Labour MP predicted the following:

> Malcolm Rifkind is not stupid, he knows concessions are necessary, and he is likely to tell Thatcher that he will not be able to implement some aspects of Tory policy such as the poll tax. ... I believe we should be laying down demands as the party that represents the people of Scotland. Rifkind needs no reminding we can create problems for him both inside and outside Parliament.
>
> (Quoted in Labour Briefing Scotland 1988: 3)

The Labour MP Brian Wilson went even further. He stated:

> No mandate exists for implementation of the poll tax in Scotland – the battle certainly cannot be won in the House of Commons alone. The government has already legislated for the introduction of the poll tax in Scotland. ... I believe that there should be a mass Scottish campaign outside Parliament to defeat the poll tax. ... the message to Mr. Rifkind that the poll tax is unenforceable can only come from the people themselves.
>
> (*The Glasgow Herald*, 17 July 1987)

However, the remodelled Labour Party, under leader Neil Kinnock, increasingly distanced itself both from the municipal left and from any forms of extra-parliamentary political activity, and there was little prospect of such fighting statements being matched by action. The 'Fighting 50' were easily kept in line and the few maverick MPs who questioned Tory authority over Scottish issues were roundly rebuked by Neil Kinnock and his Scottish lieutenant Donald Dewar (see Lavalette and Mooney 1989). As a result the Fighting 50 became known as the 'Feeble 50'. The message was clear: defeating the poll tax could not be left to parliamentary manoeuvring by Labour MPs. The Labour Party had no intention of preventing the tax from being implemented.

The 'Stop It' campaign

The 'Stop It' campaign was launched in October 1987 as a joint initiative of the Scottish Executive of the Labour Party and the STUC. The campaign was to be 'broadly based', reflecting all shades of opposition within Scotland. Its stated aim was to influence public opinion (a rather meek aim given the overwhelming opposition to the tax). It soon became apparent that the 'Stop It' campaign would operate only within the confines of existing law. Brian Wilson became chairperson of the campaign, but he dropped his previous commitment to extra-parliamentary activity and went on to become a chief spokesperson for Labour's attack on civil disobedience. Wilson got out of his embarrassing about-face with a wonderful turn of sophistry:

> [Our] aim ... should not be to advise people what to do when the Poll Tax bills come through the door – our aim ... [is] to stop them coming through the door.
>
> (Quoted in Labour Briefing Scotland 1988: 36)

Precisely how Labour was going to 'Stop It' was never addressed. A few Labour Party members duly appeared on some street corners petitioning against the tax, but in essence very little was heard from the campaign until the Scottish Labour Party Conference in March 1988. The Labour Party's inertia contrasted sharply with the expectations of Labour Party members in Scotland. The conference was inundated with demands and resolutions about how to fight the tax, and speakers denounced the Labour leadership for their inactivity and demanded that the Party commit itself to fight the tax by extra-parliamentary means. In the face of this criticism, the leadership proposed and won (thanks mainly to the union block vote) a special conference for October 1988 to be held in Govan, Glasgow. The choice of Govan was a significant one. A by-election was due in the Labour stronghold in November and the Party wanted to show how seriously it took the poll tax issue. At the re-called conference the leadership gained a significant victory for their view that the campaign must remain within the law. Less than a month later the Scottish National Party (SNP) had won a spectacular victory in Govan at the by-election and the 'Stop It' campaign had been re-launched under the financial and organizational control of the STUC.

The aim of 'Stop It' was now much clearer: it was to make the tax unworkable. With this aim the campaign asked people to return their poll tax registration forms with a series of questions. This would, they claimed, clog up the machinery and, at the very least, delay implementation. However, while the Labour Party was claiming that the poll tax would be an administrative nightmare for the government, the Regional Councils (overwhelmingly Labour dominated) and COSLA (Confederation of Scottish Local Authorities, again Labour dominated) were doing everything within their powers to ensure that the machinery for collecting the tax was in place. Indeed, Strathclyde Regional Council, which included Glasgow – and which was the largest local authority in Europe at the time – took the decision not to defy the law and to make provision for collecting the tax before the Act came into force and before either the Scottish Executive of the Labour Party or COSLA had had meetings to discuss their strategy to defeat the tax. Lothian Region (including Edinburgh) was the last regional authority to agree to implement the tax in October 1987, eighteen months before the tax was due to be implemented.

Thus, at the heart of the Labour Party's campaign was a contradiction. On the one hand, the main argument presented by the Stop It campaign was that the tax was unworkable. On the other hand, the Party's commitment to working within the law and operating as a recognised, responsible and legitimate political opposition, at both national and regional government levels, meant that Labour councils actively sought to facilitate the smooth introduction of the tax.

The 'Can Pay Won't Pay' campaign

The Scottish National Party raised the possibility of non-payment at the launch of their campaign against the poll tax at the end of 1987. Their aim was to get 100,000 people in Scotland who could pay the tax to refuse to do so on a point of principle. As well as pointing out the inequities of the tax, the SNP tapped into, and in turn fed, a growing feeling of nationalism. The introduction of the tax a year ahead of the rest of Britain, the failure of the 'Feeble 50' to defend the interests of the Scottish working class, the *perceived* existence of a North–South divide, and the fact that the SNP were at least promising to fight the government, produced one of the most dramatic by-election results of the post-war period in Scotland: their candidate Jim Sillars won Govan with a huge majority.

However, despite their apparent willingness to break the law, the SNP in Angus District (which they controlled) pressed ahead with implementation of the tax. Similarly, a split in the SNPs ranks in Grampian Region ensured that the council voted to implement a policy of wage arrestments, warrant sales and fines against those who refused to pay the tax. In the run-up to the May 1988 local elections, Alex Salmond, leader of the SNP, claimed that the SNP would lead a non-payment campaign as long as the electors wanted it, all they had to do was vote SNP to let Alex know their wishes! Finally, throughout the campaign they failed to produce their 100,000 'can but won't pay' volunteers.

The SNP's campaign was stuck within a nationalist framework. Little was said about the tax as it applied to England and Wales. For the SNP the depiction of the tax as an English Tory attack on the Scottish people was one which best matched their political aspirations, but as noted above, the Scottish middle and upper classes had been significant 'voices' demanding the new tax, keen to pursue their class interests over those of Scottish workers. Their campaign was constructed to produce a committed fighting cadre of relatively affluent Scots who would lead and win the campaign for the whole nation. By the end of the first year, as the fight spread to England and Wales, the SNP's position was undermined by the forcefulness of the response from English and Welsh non-payers.

Committees of 100

The aim of the Committees of 100 was to organize groups of 100 people who would pledge not to pay the poll tax. The initial aim of the movement was to have 'increasing circles' of committees. The initiative to set up the campaign came from a number of left Labour MPs, councillors and trade union officials within Scotland. It was a clear response to the SNP's campaign and a recognition that 'Stop It' was not engaging with the anger against the tax in the working-class districts of Scotland. The committees aimed to capture the pledge of a number of prominent MPs that they would not pay the tax. Early signatories included George Galloway, Denis Canavan and Robin Cook. Invitations were offered to representatives of other political parties, academics, clergy and trade union leaders to 'take the pledge'. However, it was made clear that these people were on the committees as 'individuals' and not as representatives of the labour or trade union movement in Scotland. Indeed, the non-involvement of large numbers of people was portrayed as a positive boon. It was argued that the mass campaign of non-payment was putting vulnerable 'poor people' at risk and also undermining the financial base of the Labour controlled councils. Thus the principled stand of a few 'leaders' could make the political gesture and gain the victory for all. Despite an initial flurry of activity, the Committees of 100 campaign did not gain widespread popular support. The setting-up of the committees in 1989 occurred at a time when the mass campaign of non-payment had been underway for nearly two years.

The linking theme in each of the above campaigns is their unswerving commitment to a tradition of 'politics from above'. In each campaign, the aim was to involve a minority of the population, or a small group of 'leaders' in political activity on behalf of the vast majority who, by definition, should passively abstain from political activity. The APTUs, however, were based on a different perspective, their aim was mass non-payment, and they tried to involve as many people in the campaign against the tax as possible.

The Anti-Poll Tax Unions

The largest and most important campaign was that organized around the APTUs: the campaign of mass non-payment. Non-payers were the most determined opponents of the tax. The tax meant a decline in living standards for most working-class families; the struggle to make ends meet for this sector of society became more difficult and, for many, paying the bill meant cutting something from the family budget. The increased cost and the effects it was having on family life meant that many working-class families came to a perfectly rational decision: 'can't pay, won't pay'. APTUs were set-up in most of the major working-class housing estates across Scotland. One of the first to be established was in Maryhil in Glasgow in April 1987. The Maryhil APTU visited houses in the area arguing against the tax and by January 1988 they had 2,000 members (Burns 1992: 29).

The aim of the APTUs was to mobilize as many people as possible and in this sense their traditions were completely different to those of the other campaigns against the tax. The priority was mass involvement based on the idea that working-class people could actively shape and direct the political process, that they were legitimate 'collective actors' who were best placed to make and meet their own needs and demands. As opposed to the other campaigns, this was a campaign organized, led and orchestrated from below.

The initial organization was undertaken by political activists in the community, many of whom were trade unionists and members of revolutionary and socialist political organizations. Some had a long history in various community and housing struggles while others were former activists who had lapsed into inactivity but became politically revitalized by the iniquitous tax and the campaign against it. Activists met in community halls or even front rooms and from there arranged meetings in their local communities. They were nearly always taken aback by the response. In apparently 'demoralized' working-class communities which had suffered from unemployment, poverty and deprivation, and within which the struggle for daily survival was immense, there were mass meetings of between 200 and 500 people, all of whom were bitterly opposed to the poll tax and were determined to fight it. The consequence was that across Scotland the APTUs' window-poster proclaiming 'No Poll Tax Here' dominated. Printed on the reverse of the poster were a list of telephone numbers of local contacts and the regional APTU office, as well as basic advice informing people what to do if they were threatened by the authorities. There were regular meetings, large and small, on estates of all sizes. The meetings informed people of the state of the campaign, organized local activities and fund-raising events and argued for new layers of people to get involved and take a lead in their locality: to spread the breadth and depth of the campaign. Tommy Sheridan, at the time a leading figure in the All Britain Anti-Poll Tax Federation and now a Scottish Socialist Party MSP in the Scottish Parliament, looking back at the early days of the campaign in Pollok, Glasgow notes that: 'We built the union through street meetings ... bus stops, traffic islands, shops, patches of spare ground all provided impromptu venues' (1994: 50).

The APTUs initially argued that people should not register for the tax. However, they soon changed strategy as it became clear that the fines for non-registration could be substantial. Instead, the APTUs developed on an organizational level forming themselves into regional networks and then a national network, and committed to a strategy of mass non-payment of the tax. Demonstrations were held in most towns and cities and demands were placed on local Labour parties and unions not to collect the tax. Nevertheless, at the heart of the campaign was a commitment to mass non-payment.

In March 1989, 15,000 people marched through Glasgow against the tax and in favour of non-payment: under the banner of the Anti-Poll Tax Federation the mass campaign of non-payment was mushrooming. On 1 April 1989 the first bills started to drop on to mats across Scotland and the extensive network of APTUs started to ensure people felt confident enough to refuse to pay. Initially there was a three-month period when little happened. No reminders were even to be sent until 'payers' were three months in arrears. By the beginning of July 1989, however, it became clear that the campaign had mobilized a substantial number of people across the country. The APTUs now moved to ensure that they could defend non-payers from attack by Sheriff Officers attempting to carry out warrant sales (the seizure and selling off by the authorities of an individual's property), wage or benefit arrestment or freezing of bank accounts (in Scotland people could not be gaoled for non-payment). The various Federations organized legal advice and helplines for non-payers and made a bold commitment – there would be no warrant sales in Scotland. The pledge was tested early, in July 1989, in Rutherglen (Glasgow) when Sheriffs threatened to 'poind' (confiscate to sell) the goods of a woman fined for non-registration. Over 300 supporters turned up to prevent the Sheriffs gaining entry to her home (Sheridan 1994: 114). To ensure these pledges could be maintained required a high level of active participation in the campaign. Telephone trees were set-up in each community so the approach of a Sheriff Officer could be met with an immediate response and the regular meetings continued to inform and organize the opposition.

The campaign went through various peaks and troughs during its first year, but non-payment was substantial and this caused immense problems for both local and national government. It is impossible to provide exact figures for non-payment, but at the end of the first year of the tax in Scotland there were two competing estimates. First, COSLA estimated that 850,000 people had not paid the tax, this number comprised of 450,000 who were subject to Court Warrant and 400,000 who were in receipt of final notices (and were thus *at least* three months behind in payment) (*Scotland on Sunday*, 1 April 1990). This represented 22 per cent of eligible payers and COSLA estimated it would lead to an 'income write-off level' of 25 per cent. But these figures were for Scotland as a whole and they hide significant geographical variation. Thus COSLA suggested that in Grampian (in the north-east of Scotland) non-payment was running at 6 per cent while in Strathclyde (which included Glasgow) 30 percent of the population had refused to pay anything at all and the Labour controlled council, far from trying to 'Stop It', had issued 300,000 summary warrants (*Scotland on Sunday*, 1 April 1990).

The second source of non-payment figures came from the Scottish Anti-Poll Tax who claimed that one million Scots had either not paid or were significantly in arrears and that non-payment in Glasgow was running at 45 per cent (*Militant*, 9 March 1990). As Tommy Sheridan notes:

> Non-payment in Scotland had become a deluge. It was like water seeping through the wall of a dam. Just a trickle at first. Then more rapid splashes through the hairline crack. These became a stream. The crack bursts open and you had a flood.
>
> (Sheridan 1994: 112)

By the end of the first year of the campaign, mass non-payment in Scotland had ensured that the APTUs had hegemony in the anti-tax movement. The levels of non-payment were astonishingly high, presenting Labour controlled local councils in Scotland and the Tory government nationally with a serious political problem. Intensifying the problem was the fact that the tax was spreading: from the 1 April 1990 the poll tax applied to the whole of Britain.

As the campaign against the tax spread it took a more visibly militant turn. By the end of March 1990 the All Britain Federation had over 1,500 affiliated unions across the country, making it a truly mass movement. As the first poll tax rates were set in the town halls across England and Wales, the APTUs held demonstrations and pickets outside council chambers. It was not just the inner cities that witnessed such demonstrations. In the south-west of England, for example, Burns (1992: 84–5) suggests that over 50,000 people attended major demonstrations, including 8,000 in Plymouth, 5,000 each in Taunton, Paignton and Exeter, 3,000 in Barnstable and 1,500 in Bath. Town halls were the scene of clashes between police and protesters in many London boroughs, as well as in Newcastle, Southampton, Norwich, Colchester and Bristol. On 6 March in Bristol, as protesters met to demonstrate against the setting of the tax rate, police snatch squads moved in to arrest a demonstrator. Burns takes up the story:

> The whole crowd turned ... and started running towards the police. People grabbed those who had been arrested and pulled

them away. The police brought in reinforcements and charged the crowd with horses.

(Burns 1992: 85)

On 7 March protesters gathered at Hackney Town Hall in London and tried to enter the council chamber to prevent councillors setting the tax rate. The crowd was charged by Metropolitan police officers wielding batons, but rather than disperse the protesters stood their ground and fought. Bottles, bricks, stones, sticks and placards rained down on the police and fighting spread up the High Street. Across England and Wales councillors setting the poll tax rate were met by demonstrations, with protesters occasionally forcing their way into council chambers. These demonstrations were usually peaceful, but sometimes they turned violent.

But where violence did occur, such confrontations were the result of two main elements. First was the anger and hostility felt by people towards the tax, and within this a general dissatisfaction with much of the Tories' economic and social agenda: the poll tax had become the focus of anger against ten years' of Tory rule. Second was the police tactics at the demonstrations. During the 1980s policing of demonstrations and industrial conflict had become increasingly brutal, most notably the attacks on the miners at Orgreave and numerous pit villages during 1984/85, and the printers and their supporters at Wapping in 1986. By 1990 the police force was treating demonstrators in a particularly 'aggressive' way, increasing tension and the likelihood of conflict.

The town hall confrontations did not stop councils setting their poll tax rates, but they did help to intensify the campaign, to give confidence to the protesters and to generate an atmosphere of hope that the tax could be beaten. They also fed a growing unease within the Tory Party with regard to the extent of opposition the tax was generating. One Tory backbencher, Tony Marlow, told the 1922 Committee that there was a danger the government could be seen to be 'declaring war on the people' (*Glasgow Herald*, 2 March 1990). In desperation, the Tory leadership attempted to blame the conflict on Labour non-paying MPs, of whom there were thirty, and the Militant Tendency in the Labour Party. Neil Kinnock, on the other hand, denounced 'toytown revolutionaries' and Roy Hattersley tried to blame the Socialist Workers Party. Despite distancing themselves from the action, however, Labour was clearly benefiting from the anti-Tory mood. Opinion polls in March 1990 emphasized how unpopular the tax and the government were, with Labour reaping the benefit (see

Table 11.2). For example, a by-election on 22 March in the safe Tory seat of Mid-Staffordshire saw Labour overturn a Tory majority of 14,000 to win by 9,000 votes.

Table 11.2   National opinion poll finding, March 1990

Poll	Labour lead over Conservatives (%)
Observer/Harris	28
Sunday Correspondent/ICM	27
Sunday Times/MORI	23

But the town hall confrontations were also vital in building support for the demonstrations against the tax to be held on 31 March 1990 in London, Glasgow and Cheltenham. These demonstrations would turn out to be the turning point in the anti-poll tax campaign. In total, the two main demonstrations attracted approximately 250,000 marchers – around 50,000 in Glasgow and 200,000 in London. The Glasgow demonstration started early in the day and was a massive show of defiance from non-payers and opponents. But it was the demonstration in London which would have the decisive effect.

Demonstrators gathered in Kennington Park in London waiting for the march to start. The park gradually filled to become a swarming mass of people, comprising old and young, men and women, black and white, gay and straight, the able-bodied and the disabled, standing together as one. There was something of a carnival atmosphere, with a number of bands playing and the park covered in banners and placards. The Labour Party and many trade unions had gone out of their way to discourage their members and branches from participating – but none the less there were Labour and trade union banners, as well as those from the Socialist Workers Party, Militant Tendency and numerous anti-poll tax groups. Perhaps the biggest cheer came when a group of ex-miners unfurled their banner: 'Miners against the Poll Tax' (*Socialist Worker*, 7 April 1990).

At 1.30 p.m. the march set off. At 3 p.m. a small sit-down protest took place outside Downing Street. The police response was brutal:

A man in a wheelchair was attacked and arrested ... separated from his wheelchair and thrown into a police van. A woman was arrested and, in front of the crowd, stripped of her clothes.

(Burns 1992: 89)

The heavy-handed tactics by police incensed the crowd and set in motion a process that led to the 'battle of Trafalgar' (Stott 1998). The battle of Trafalgar began when police attacked demonstrators in Whitehall, forcing them into Trafalgar Square. In the Square, police horses and vans were driven into the massive crowd, causing serious injury. For many in the Square, boxed in by the police, there was no alternative but to fight. But this time, unlike many of the big confrontations between the police and protesters during the 1980s, the anti-poll tax protesters were able to resist the police assaults. The police were beaten back and the crowd pushed out beyond the Square. The South African Embassy, the symbol of apartheid in the heart of London, was set on fire as were various shops and cars lining the escape routes. But the violence was not random: the targets were the symbols of Thatcherism. Corner shops and vendors' stands were left unharmed; it was the shops and cars of the rich that were attacked. As Sheridan notes:

> The rampage was not entirely indiscriminate. ... They smashed the windows of Porsches. They overturned BMWs ... I didn't hear of too many Ladas being torched. Stringfellows, the uppercrust nightclub, was wrecked but the pub next door was untouched.
>
> (Sheridan 1994: 128)

The aftermath of the protests left the Tories reeling and in the international press it was taken to signify a great malaise at the heart of Thatcher's Britain.

The state took a hard line in response to the protests. Over 300 people were arrested on the day of the march and in the weeks that followed police across the country were involved in Operation Carnaby which produced a further 150 arrests. Some police used this opportunity to harass local activists. The trials of the accused did not always go in favour of the police. The Trafalgar Square Defence Committee (TSDC), which was set up in the aftermath of the battle of Trafalgar to offer legal advice and help to those arrested, had some success in the courts. (TSDC was set up independently from the Federation due to two leading members denouncing those who had been arrested.) On many occasions juries found in favour of the accused. In one notable case, the defendant:

> a student and ex-miner, was cleared of Violent Disorder after claiming he had acted in self-defence in order to protect the crowd

from police baton charges. He admitted in open court that he had thrown missiles at the police and was shown on video doing so.

(Burns 1992: 115)

In other instances, TSDC was able to question and undermine police evidence. For example, in a case heard at Southwark Crown Court in 1991 TSDC argued that the main prosecution witness, PC Carre-Brown, could not have witnessed the events which he claimed to have seen unless he was able to see *through* the South African Embassy (in the event, the judge threw out the case) (Mitchell 1998).

However, some protesters were given heavy prison sentences and in subsequent months a large number of people were gaoled for non-payment. But the battle of Trafalgar marked the beginning of the end. In opinion polls conducted after the battle, it was clear the majority of people blamed the Tories and the poll tax for the 'riot': as Margaret Thatcher bitterly admitted, 'law-abiding, decent people' had gone over to 'the mob' (1993: 661). In the May council elections Labour became the benefactors of the anti-Tory mood and gained over 300 seats. The tactic of non-payment continued and the APTUs turned to full-scale defence of those facing charges and wage arrestment. In court, self-taught union activists provided defence for non-payers. On several occasions courtrooms were stormed by protesters, and non-payers appeared *en masse* to clog up the proceedings. The administrative and political nightmare the Tories had created continued.

The government persevered with the tax but anti-poll tax pressure was building in the Tory Party, with such prominent Tories as Geoffrey Howe, Nigel Lawson and Michael Heseltine attacking the policy and Thatcher's governmental style. In November 1990 Thatcher suffered a leadership challenge instigated by the poll tax issue. Although she won the vote, she failed to obtain an overall majority. On the 20 November Thatcher resigned as prime minister, sunk by the poll tax.

John Major became the new prime minister and although he initially claimed the tax would remain, the administrative nightmare and the by-election result in the Ribble Valley in March 1991 – where the Liberal Democrats won a solid Tory seat – changed everything. Michael Heseltine was instructed to produce an alternative tax. The poll tax had been consigned to the dustbin of history.

Class and community: the nature of the anti-poll tax movement

The APTM gained hegemony within the poll tax opposition because it engaged directly with the vast majority who opposed the tax and whose standard of living would be detrimentally affected by its imposition. But what was the nature of the APTM? There has been some suggestion from academics that the APTMs represented a 'community'-based 'new social movement' as opposed to a 'class' movement. For example, Tonge stresses the 'broad-based, mass movement, with decentralised, non-hierarchical organisational forms which appeared characteristic of a social movement' (1995: 1). While Hoggett and Burns stress the 'community-based' nature of the anti-poll tax protests:

> Its true legacy is surely that a mass campaign was built which reached into the heart of communities. In many areas it completely restored the whole idea of community and collective organisation. The community alone ... took on the Thatcher Government and won, demonstrating the power it can wield if it develops a collective consciousness.
>
> (1991: 109)

Other commentators have suggested it was the revolt of 'middle England' which defeated the tax. That the protests involved some groups of people who were not working class and who did not live in traditional working-class areas is evident from any serious exploration of the anti-poll tax organization (although all great working-class upsurges draw in people from other social classes or contradictory class locations within the class structure, as the power, drive and unity of the working class in these episodes opens up a wider vision of an improved world). But such developments can be overstated and many of the above claims ignore the way in which the working class has been restructured and reorganized in the post-war years to include the vast majority of white-collar workers, such as teachers, civil servants and local government workers, for example. So the claim that 'middle England' was significant often means that teachers, social workers, local government workers and nurses, to name but a few, were heavily involved in the campaign. But why should this surprise us and how does this undermine the class base of the movement?

Further, the claim that 'grass-roots' organizations 'from below' are somehow distinct from class-based organizations does not stand up to scrutiny. The chapters within this volume emphasize the range of 'grass-roots' organizations that emerge from working-class communities during periods of struggle. In addition, there are many examples of workplace disputes where the struggles and protests were not controlled by 'official' labour and trade union bodies, the leadership of which have often attempted to harness and curtail such protests (for a recent example, see Lavalette and Kennedy 1996).

The problem with those who argue for social movement over class-based protest lies in their narrow and somewhat ahistorical and deterministic approach and interpretation of working-class struggle and working-class political organization. Their overriding emphasis on 'community' – as something which remains distinct from working-class protest – is both symptomatic and a reflection of this kind of approach.

It would be wrong to say that the campaign everywhere took similar forms. But the intensity of the opposition, as reflected in large-scale non-payment rates, was clearly centred on working-class areas in urban centres across Britain. In West Central Scotland, and in Scotland's other major urban areas, together with those in the major English and Welsh cities, the anti-poll tax campaign was rooted in working-class districts, but in ways which transcended the narrow, 'keep within the law' approach of the Labour Party and trade union leadership. That millions of working men and women were prepared to defy such calls, and were prepared to look beyond the majority of labour movement organizations to organize against the poll tax, does not make them any less working class or the campaign less class-based.

Conclusion

The poll tax was introduced by the Tories as a way to push through their agenda of privatizing welfare, increasing inequality and banishing social democracy from local government. It was formed at a time when the government's confidence in its ability to face down working-class opposition knew few bounds. It had defeated the miners and the main battalions of the trade union movement, it had defeated the left-Labour councils and the Labour leadership was distancing itself from all forms of extra-parliamentary activity. This was the government's moment and the poll tax suitably matched its ideological goals. Yet the tax generated a 'most remarkable mass movement' (Hoggett and Burns 1991: 95) which defeated the tax and led to the removal of Margaret Thatcher as prime minister. We leave the final comment to that most respectable of newspapers, the *Observer*. On the 24 March 1991, its editorial stated:

If the Poll Tax is dead it was killed by non-payment, a tactic which each of the three main parties insisted was pointless and wrong. ... Extra-Parliamentary action ... proved itself and in the process exposed the hollowness of our claims to democracy ... each and every one of those non-payers should feel proud of themselves ... it was left to ... [an] army of ordinary people to destroy a bad law.

Note

1 The split between 'economic' and 'political' conflicts is much confused and far less clear-cut than this implies. Indeed, the historic divergence between politics and economics has been one of the great weaknesses of the labour movement in Britain; for more on this subject see Cliff and Gluckstein (1988).

12   Identity politics or class struggle?

The case of the mental health users' movement.

Iain Ferguson

Introduction

Less than eight months after New Labour's landslide election victory of May 1997, a group of disabled activists, some in wheelchairs, chained themselves to the gates of Downing Street in London and threw red paint on to the gates and the road. Their actions were part of a protest against the new government's proposed review of disability benefits, a review which many disabled people feared would be a precursor to substantial cuts in their benefits. The significance of such protests was twofold. On the one hand, it provided an early indication of the anger and concern felt by many at New Labour's proposed programme of welfare reform. On the other, it pointed to the continuing growth of often militant self-organization among groups of people who for a variety of reasons are particularly dependent on the services of the welfare state. In this chapter, I wish to focus on one example of such self-organization, the mental health users' movement (MHUM). Although smaller and less visible than the disability movement, the mental health users' movement has grown significantly over the past decade.

While no single set of ideas dominates the MHUM, there is evidence in recent years of the growing influence among some user groups of *identity politics*, based on the idea that all mental health service users share a common interest which overrides any other interest or division (Aronowitz 1992). The central argument of this chapter is that such identity politics are incapable of providing a basis for challenging the stigma and material inequality experienced by the vast majority of people with mental health problems and that class-based politics provide the only firm basis for such a challenge. The argument will be presented in two parts. In the first half of the chapter

I explore the extent to which it is possible to speak of users of mental health services as 'oppressed' and to consider the nature of that oppression. In the second half, I discuss the movement of service users that has developed to oppose the stigma and discrimination which users experience. I then go on to critically evaluate its characterization by writers within the critical social policy literature as a 'new social movement' (Rogers and Pilgrim 1991; Pilgrim and Rogers 1993; Barnes and Shardlow 1996; Barnes 1997), or occasionally, 'new social welfare movement' (Williams 1992). These terms are sometimes used in a *descriptive* sense (to suggest that the movement in practice is more concerned with cultural than material issues, for example) and sometimes in a *prescriptive* sense (to imply a particular strategic direction for service users wishing to challenge their oppression). Finally, I shall argue that the classical Marxist analysis of oppression, rather than the analyses offered by 'identity politics' which draw on conceptions of postmodernity, provides the most fruitful basis both for an understanding of the specific nature of the oppression of people with mental health problems and also for developing a strategy for challenging that oppression.

Before proceeding, a brief note on terminology is necessary. There is no agreed term within the mental health users' movement for people who use mental health services, with terms such as user, service user, survivor and even mad person being used. At one level, such debates are a frequent and perhaps necessary feature of the emergence of any new movement. On the other, they can become a substitute for addressing more difficult issues, such as how to defend community-based services, and can lead to a high level of internalization. In this chapter, I shall employ the term 'user' or 'service user', both for the sake of consistency and also because it is still the most widely used term, while acknowledging that many people with mental health problems strongly object to the term.

Mental ill-health and oppression

While the disability movement has had some success in recent years in winning the argument that 'disability' is often socially constructed, rather than being the inevitable product of mental or physical impairment (Barton 1996; Oliver 1996; Oliver and Barnes 1998), the continuing dominance of the biomedical model of mental health means that many of the problems experienced by people with mental health problems, such as poverty, unemployment and social isolation, are still more likely to be seen as the 'natural' consequence of mental ill-health. Yet while mental health problems clearly *do* impair the functioning of people experiencing them, structural factors are often at least as significant, and sometimes more so. In this section, three aspects of such structural oppression will be examined: the impact of stigma; the medical model of mental illness; and exclusion from the labour market.

Stigma

The starting point for any examination of the experience of people with mental health problems is an acknowledgement of the all-pervading stigma which they experience. Reviewing the American experience, for example, Warner has argued that:

> It is obvious that mental patients are still highly stigmatised. Branded as 'psychos' in popular parlance, they encounter great hardship in finding employment and generate fear as to their dangerousness. Citizens fight to exclude psychiatric treatment facilities and living quarters for the mentally ill from their neighbourhoods. The status afforded the mentally ill is the very lowest.
>
> (Warner 1994: 180)

In most respects, the picture in Britain is similar to the one in the States. A recent national survey of the views of mental health workers by the Health Education Authority (1998), for example, found that the two most common reasons given by their patients for experiencing discrimination were being labelled mentally ill and racism. Another general population survey carried out by the Scottish Association for Mental Health (1998) found that 48 per cent of those interviewed concurred with the statement that 'If I was suffering mental health problems, I wouldn't want anyone to know about it'.

It could perhaps be argued that such attitudes towards people with mental health problems reflect a realistic perception of the danger that they pose to other members of society, but this argument does not stand up to serious examination. The conclusion of one of several major reports into the danger posed by people with mental health problems living in the community was that public fear of random killings by such individuals is based on myth (*Guardian*, 12 December 1997). The research, carried out for the Department of Health at Manchester University, found that arbitrary attacks are rare. People are almost three times more likely to be killed by a stranger who is not mentally ill than one who is. Of 408 homicide convictions in one year, only 12 per cent were carried out by people who 'had been in contact with mental health services' during the twelve months preceding their offence, with the overwhelming majority of homicides by mentally ill people involving not strangers but family members. By contrast, over 1,000 people with mental health problems are likely to kill themselves each year. Very similar findings were arrived at by the Boyd Inquiry, set-up by a previous government in the wake of a number of homicides involving people with mental health problems (*Confidential Inquiry* 1994).

All such homicides are tragic. But as Larkin (1994) argues, what they tend to highlight, however, is less the dangerousness of people with mental health problems than the chronic under-resourcing of mental health services. It is, however, the issue of dangerousness and not resources that is emphasized both in the media and in social policy discussion. Among the findings of the Boyd Inquiry for example were the following: that less than one homicide a month involves someone with mental health problems; that a quarter of these involved the killing of small children by depressed mothers; that three-quarters of the thirty-four individuals involved were felt to be receiving the appropriate level of support and supervision by professionals involved with them; that very few had defaulted on their medication; and that only a third had a diagnosis of schizophrenia. Despite this, these findings were reported in the popular press with such headlines as 'One murder a fortnight by mentally ill' (*Daily Telegraph*, 17 August 1994), 'Scandal of loonies freed to kill' (*Daily Star*, 18 August 1994) and 'Free to kill' (*The Sun*, 18 August 1994) (Crepaz-Keay 1996).

The fact that it is the alleged dangerousness of people with mental health problems that forms the central theme of both media and government concern suggests a process of scapegoating is at work, one effect of which is to divert attention away from the lack of services for people with mental health problems. More generally, constructing mental ill-health in this way has profound consequences for the development of policies and services (Saraga 1998). At an informal level, it leads to the exclusion of people with mental health problems from employment, housing and many areas of social contact; at a social policy level, it has led in recent years to an emphasis on the need to *control* the behaviour of people with mental health problems, with such control usually involving an emphasis on the taking of powerful medication and greater compulsion in the community, rather than a focus on the factors which create or worsen mental health problems in the first place and the kind of services that could reduce mental distress.

The biomedical model of mental ill-health

A second aspect of the oppression of people with mental health problems relates to the dominance of the biomedical model of mental ill-health. At the heart of this model is the notion that such ill-health is an 'illness', in essence no different from physical illness, the roots of which lie in biology rather than in social factors and in response to which physical treatments, in the form of drugs, ECT, or even brain surgery, constitute the first, if not the only, course of action.

The dominance of this model is a reflection of three main factors. First, there is the 150-year-old professional and institutional hegemony of the psychiatric profession over all matters relating to mental distress (Busfield 1986). Different psychiatrists, of course, will vary in the role that they attribute to biological factors, and there is evidence that in general British psychiatrists are more willing to consider the role of social factors than their American counterparts (Rowe 1993). Nevertheless, an acceptance of the *primary* role of biological factors in the aetiology of mental ill-health continues to characterize most psychiatric practice. Underpinning and reinforcing this dominance is the power of the pharmaceutical companies. For example, Prozac is prescribed to more than 10 million people world-wide and its sales run to over \$1.3 billion annually (Breggin and Breggin 1995). A casual glance at the advertisements in any issue of the *British Journal of Psychiatry* vividly illustrates the role played by these companies in framing psychiatric responses to problems of mental ill-health.

A second factor contributing to the dominance of psychiatry in matters relating to mental health is the *ideological* role played by psychiatry in individualizing mental distress and deflecting attention away from the role of structural factors both in the production of mental ill-health and in responses to it. The fact, for example, that working-class women with children are four times more likely to experience clinical depression than their middle-class counterparts is obscured by seeing depression as primarily an individual or biological problem (Brown and Harris 1978). Similarly, the over-representation of black people at the coercive end of the psychiatric system is well-documented (Littlewood and Lipsedge 1989; Fernando 1995).

Finally, there is the fact, neglected by some radical critiques of psychiatry, that in some respects at least, mental ill-health *does* resemble physical illness, both at a philosophical level (Sedgewick 1982) and in terms of its impact on social functioning. In his study of psychiatry and political economy, for example, the Marxist psychiatrist Richard Warner, argues that:

Schizophrenia ... fulfils any criteria we might wish to establish to define an illness. It is a non-volitional and generally maladaptive condition which decreases the person's functional capacity and which may be identified by a reasonably circumscribed set of characteristic features.

(Warner 1994: 4)

Given the growing dominance on both sides of the Atlantic of 'Third Way' perspectives which emphasize the 'employability' of disabled citizens as a means of reducing welfare benefits and coercing individuals back into the workforce (Blair 1998), the recognition that mental ill-health is often disabling and incapacitating needs to be stressed, alongside the need to challenge the discrimination that keeps those who have experienced mental health problems out of the workforce. It is this dimension of mental ill-health that social constructionist perspectives often fail to grasp. Yet as Barham and Hayward comment:

If ... there is a form of medical reductionism which quickly disposes of the whole struggle to get to grips with the other person, then there is also an opposing form of normalising discourse in which difference comes to be glossed over or denied, as though a benign regard or the force of good intentions could prose away the stubborn reality of chronic mental illness.

(Barham and Hayward 1995: 5)

Exclusion from the labour market

A third aspect of the oppression of people with mental health problems is their exclusion from the labour market. A survey carried out in the mid-1980s found that where work applicants demonstrated equal experience and training employers discriminated against those who 'confessed' to having had a mental health problem at some time in the past (cited in Rogers *et al.* 1993). In part, this is linked to the stigma discussed above. This was one topic covered in a recent series of interviews which I conducted with activists in the MHUM in Scotland. As one respondent said:

I fill in application forms and if it says, 'are you suffering from depression?', I lie. I mean, I wouldn't admit to that because I feel I would be put right down the bottom of the heap. It's just there, you know, it still has the stigma. I don't care what anybody says, there is a certain amount of stigma attached to mental illness.

There is considerable evidence that given proper support, many people with histories of mental health problems are capable of maintaining employment. The success of the clubhouse model of rehabilitation (Mastboom 1992), for example, based on Fountain House in New York and with an emphasis on transitional employment schemes, attests to the employment potential of people with mental health problems (Oliver *et al.* 1996). The argument that it is social, economic and political factors rather than impairment *per se* that affects the employment prospects of people with mental health problems is also supported by research evidence. On the basis of a review of the research literature on employment and mental health, Warner has argued that there is a relationship between the booms and slumps of the capitalist economy on the one hand and the employment of people with mental health problems on the other. Higher recovery rates occur during periods of economic upturn, which suggests that when there is a shortage of labour, there is a much more positive attitude towards employing former patients. Hence his definition of schizophrenia as 'an illness which is shaped, to a large extent, by political economy' (1994: 1).

The strength of Warner's argument is that, without ignoring or downplaying the often devastating impact of mental ill-health, he sees the problems of poverty and social isolation experienced by people with mental health problems not as the inevitable consequences of mental ill-health but rather as the consequence of a particular social and economic order. In similar vein, Sedgewick argues that any strategy for mental health services

> must come, above all, from the realisation that some of the most basic needs of the mentally disabled – above all, the needs for housing, for occupation and for community – are not satisfied by the market system of allocation which operates under capitalism. … The crisis of mental-health provision … is simply the crisis of the normal social order in relation to any of its members who lack the wage-based ticket of entry into its palace of commodities.
>
> (Sedgewick 1982: 239)

What this suggests is that while mental health problems may from time to time affect an individual's ability to maintain employment, stigmatizing attitudes on the part of employers, a lack of supported employment schemes and the demands on the labour process within capitalism (which, in the form of stress, affect far larger numbers of workers than those labelled as mentally ill) are more significant factors.

The above discussion of the impact of stigma, of the role of the biomedical model of mental health and of the effects of exclusion from the labour market strongly suggests that many of the problems experienced by people with mental health problems cannot be seen as the 'natural' consequences of poor mental health but rather are often the product of structural discrimination and oppression. I shall argue below that this oppression differs in important respects from the oppression suffered by black people and women. It is none the less real and it is at least in part in response to this discrimination and oppression that the current mental health users' movement has developed over the past fifteen years or so (Barnes 1997). It is to a consideration of this movement that we shall now turn.

Mental health service users – a 'new social movement'?

While the nature of the mental health users' movement makes it difficult to estimate the actual numbers of users or former users involved, one activist has estimated that the number of user groups has grown from around a dozen in the mid-1980s to around 350 nation-wide by the mid-1990s (Campbell 1996). Not all of these groups are campaigning groups. In her account of the movement, Lindow classifies them as *reactive* (advocacy projects, campaigning organizations), *alternative* (crisis centres, user-controlled projects) and *creative* (including Hearing Voices groups or Survivors' Poetry) (Lindow 1995). What is likely to characterize all, or most of them, however, is the active involvement of users or former users in activities which to some degree challenge dominant, negative stereotypes of people with mental health problems.

This involvement of users or former users is one feature which distinguishes the current movement from earlier mental health movements, such as the anti-psychiatry movement of the late 1960s and early 1970s, based on the ideas and activities of R. D. Laing. As Kotowicz has noted, while Laing and his colleagues in the 1960s may have given people with schizophrenia a 'voice', British anti-psychiatry (in contrast to radical mental health movements elsewhere, such as Italy) was based very much on a small number of radical psychiatrists and other professionals, with little if any involvement by patients themselves (with the Mental Health Patients' Union, for example, only being set-up in 1973) (Kotowicz 1997).

The involvement of numbers of users in challenging the discrimination and oppression experienced by users is also a factor which has led some academic writers who are sympathetic to the movement to conceptualize it as a 'new social movement' (NSM), similar to the gay movement or the women's movement. Barnes and Shardlow, for example, have argued that 'A potentially useful sociological perspective which we are starting to apply ... is that of new social movement theory' (1996: 130). While Pilgrim and Rogers take the position that:

> user dissatisfaction has now reached a point that, in terms of numbers and organisations, it constitutes a nascent 'new social movement'. Social movements can be defined as certain groups engaged in informal efforts in order to promote their interests in opposition to dominant forms of power and organisation preferred by the State. ... 'New' social movements can be distinguished conceptually from 'old' social movements in that they are further removed from the arena of production than the latter. Additionally, rather than seeking to defend existing social and property rights from erosion by the state, they seek to establish new agendas and conquer new territory.
>
> (Pilgrim and Rogers 1993: 173)

In so far as describing mental health users as a social movement refers to the development of *collective* organization among users and to their involvement in activities which to some degree at least are *oppositional* in nature, the term seems appropriate and unobjectionable. One leading social movement theorist, for example, has argued that:

> The proper analogy for a social movement is neither a party nor a union but a political campaign. What we call a social movement consists in a series of demands of challenges to power-holders in the name of a social category that lacks an established political position.
>
> (Tilly, cited in Foweraker 1995: 80)

The extent to which users can and do challenge power-holders will be considered more fully below. But the characterization of the users' movement as a *new* social movement has a different, more contentious meaning. First, it implies a preoccupation with issues of *identity*, which

Foweraker identifies as the defining feature of new social movement theory (Foweraker 1995). Second, it suggests a focus on *cultural* or *ideological* issues rather than material issues. Third, it implies that *class-based* politics have limited relevance in challenging the discrimination and oppression experienced by users. What are the implications of each of these themes?

Identity issues

In respect of identity, there is little doubt that personal experience, rather than an altruistic concern with the issue of mental ill-health, is the most common reason for people becoming involved in the mental health users' movement. Barnes and Shardlow, for example, note that:

> Our research suggests that the factors which provide the strongest motivation to participate in mental health user groups are the shared experiences of distress and of being a recipient of mental health services – of being a 'patient'.
>
> (Barnes and Shardlow 1996: 130)

In similar vein, the single most important feature of the MHUM identified by Rogers and Pilgrim and described by them as ' "the" identifying characteristic of the users' movement in Britain' (1991: 135), was an emphasis on the *experience* of being a psychiatric patient and the need for that experience to be recognized and validated. This finding is reinforced both by the subsequent, and much more extensive research conducted by Rogers, Pilgrim and Lacey (1993) as well as by the writings of users such as Sassoon and Lindow (1995), who emphasize 'the validation of the user's view'.

Two points can be made about this basis for involvement. On the one hand, given the stigma and social isolation experienced by people with mental health problems, the existence of a movement or at least of groups of people who have been through similar experiences and who are able to recognize and validate each other's experience can be an enormously important source of confidence and social support.

That said, while experience may provide an initial basis for involvement, by itself it does not lead to the development of a strategy for challenging oppression, a point noted by both Rogers and Pilgrim (1991) and Barnes and Shardlow (1996). In part, this is because experience is necessarily subjective and not all users share the same experience, any more than the physically impaired do. Challenging the notion that all disabled people share a common identity, for example,

Stack, in discussing the disability movement from a Marxist perspective, has argued that:

> As with all movements of the oppressed, there is a class basis to it. If Rupert Murdoch had a disabled child, that child would face very few obstacles in its life compared not just to me or working class disabled people but to most able bodied people.
>
> (Stack 1995: 15)

Class is also a major division among mental health service users. Not only do the politicians, businesspeople and celebrities who pay £3,000 a week to have their mental health problems treated at the private Priory group of hospitals, for example, enjoy forms of care and treatment beyond the wildest dreams of most people who become mentally unwell (*Observer*, 1 October 1999), but they are also unlikely to experience the day to day concerns and worries of having to survive on benefits or of struggling to access either acute psychiatric services or patchy and under-resourced community-based services which is the fate of most service users. Nor is there much evidence that it has a profound or lasting effect on lifestyle or career prospects, in contrast to the kind of employment discrimination experienced by poorer service users discussed above.

Yet while there has been a growing recognition within the literature in recent years of the relationship between mental ill-health and 'race' on the one hand (Fernando 1995) and mental ill-health and women's oppression on the other (Busfield 1996), the profound impact of class differences at every stage of the process of mental ill-health has often been neglected, even in the more radical literature. Thus, for example, as Sedgewick has noted, *Social Class and Mental Illness*, the pioneering work by Hollingshead and Redlich published in the late 1950s which looked at the ways in which a person's social class affected the kind of psychiatric treatment he/she received, was completely ignored by all the major anti-psychiatric writers (1982: 278). Far from all people with mental health problems sharing a common experience, however, every aspect of mental ill-health from its inception to its treatment is coloured by class. As Gomm has noted:

> A very simple statement will serve to summarise all the research findings on this matter: for nearly, every kind of disease, illness or disability, 'physical' and 'mental', poorer people are afflicted more than richer people; more often, more seriously and for longer –

unless of course they die from the condition, which they do at an earlier age.

(Gomm 1996: 110)

Thus, as noted above, a key finding of the classic study of depression by Brown and Harris (1978) was that working-class women with children were four times more likely to experience depression than their middle-class counterparts. In respect of schizophrenia, a recent report by the Child Poverty Action Group states that schizophrenia is diagnosed five times more often in low socio-economic status adolescents compared with high socio-economic status adolescents – in other words, before 'social drift' may have occurred. In respect of unemployment, a 1993 study found that the unemployment rate is the most effective predictor of psychiatric admission (Henderson *et al.* 1998).

To stress the importance of class and other structural factors such as 'race' and gender, is not, of course, to deny the possibility that biological factors may play a predisposing role in the development of certain psychotic conditions, as Warner argues, let alone in organic conditions such as epilepsy or Alzheimer's disease (Warner 1994). Nor is it to ignore the obvious fact that mental ill-health affects individuals from all classes. It does mean, however, that not only are poor and working-class people more likely to suffer from mental ill-health but that the implications of being mentally ill are much more severe. The centrality of *material* issues for most service users was one of the major conclusions of the study of 516 service users carried out by Roger, Pilgrim and Lacey:

> If users' views reported in this book were replicated and implemented at the level of policy, then the current emphasis on physical 'treatments' would be drastically reduced. It would be replaced by two types of professional activity: the first would be in terms of being listened to and responded to empathetically ... the second would be in terms of the recognition of the centrality of social needs. ... Given that recovery from mental health problems is a function of social opportunities, particularly as regards accommodation and employment, policy-makers might place housing and income maintenance at the centre of their thoughts.
>
> (Roger *et al.* 1993: 183–4)

This point bears directly on the two other elements of NSM politics referred to earlier, namely, on the one hand, the alleged emphasis on cultural and ideological issues rather than material issues, and on the other, the supposed irrelevance of class politics.

Cultural and ideological issues.

It is clear that material issues *do* loom large in the lives of the majority of service users. If then, the groups researched by Pilgrim and Rogers on one hand and Barnes and Shardlow on the other fail to address these issues, is it possible that an emphasis on cultural or ideological issues is a *contingent* rather than an essential feature of the users' movement? My own research into the users' movement in Scotland suggests that this may in fact be the case. In the study of nine user-led projects and five other user groups across central Scotland, involving over eighty users, it was clear that the groups were involved in a range of campaigning activities. Many of these campaigns were clearly around 'material' issues. Thus, for example, members of the Fife Survivors' Group (whose names have been changed to protect confidentiality) had organized letter-writing campaigns around a wide variety of issues (even if the results were not always what they hoped):

George: We've written several letters to MPs in Fife about various issues such as psychosurgery, the loss of the mobility component in DLA [Disabled Living Allowance] where people are in hospital so they haven't been in care.

Anne: We did write to all the councillors this time last year on the service cuts to the voluntary sector … all councillors got a letter and we wrote to the *Scotsman*, the *Courier* and various papers … the local papers printed it, the *Scotsman* and the *Courier* didn't … of course the response from the council was very poor. There were maybe two who replied eventually and the leader of the council replied.

Moreover, some of the groups, including Edinburgh Users' Forum, had been involved in more public campaigning activities, including demonstrations, particularly around the substantial cuts in Scottish local authority and voluntary organizations spending which took place in 1997.

Kate: In the past year, we've been involved in quite a few campaigns, some small, some big. I think the biggest one we did was the cuts campaign, against the local council cuts in services. That was actually quite a big campaign as it in-

volved other agencies and we were all quite exhausted at
the end of it, the workers as well.

Jack: We were in contact with old age pensioners, UNISON, and
all sorts of other groups ...

Kate: ... who were also being threatened by the cuts basically.
That was the joint march on the 1 March through Edinburgh and then some of them went off to a rally but then
we organized and chaired a meeting at the South Side
Community Centre to which those other people were in-
vited but we did a lot of work before that on our own,
writing to MPs, local councillors, a deputation to the council – that was sort of the biggest thing we did. We did a lot
of smaller things.

That campaigning was not confined to one or two groups was
evident at the Scottish Users' Conference in February 1997 where a
well-attended workshop was held on the topic 'How to fight the cuts',
attended by members of groups from several parts of Scotland. For
those who can afford private mental health care, whether in the form
of psychotherapy or of private providers such as the Priory hospitals,
such cuts are unlikely to have much impact on their day to day lives.
For the majority of users, however, they can make the difference
between an existence in which there is the possibility of fellowship,
solidarity and change on the one hand and a lonely and frightening
isolation on the other.

Something else is suggested, however, by the above examples,
namely the possibility of common ground with trade unions,
community groups and other disabled organizations around issues
such as the defence of community-based services and opposition to
council cuts. It is precisely the possibility of such alliances that NSM
theory and identity politics often deny and to the discussion of which
we now turn.

A politics of identity?

A core tenet of new social movement theory, reinforced by the
assumptions of postmodernism, is that not only do all members of an
oppressed group share a common interest and identity (overriding all
other divisions, such as class) but also that the primary responsibility
for challenging that oppression lies with the members of that group.
As Smith has argued in a critique of 'new social movement' analyses:

Key to this strategy for social change, which has been carried to its logical extreme more recently through the development of 'identity politics', is the idea that only those experiencing a particular form of oppression can either define it or fight against it.

(Smith 1994: 3)

In an example of such identity politics, Mike Oliver, a leading disability theorist and activist, has argued that 'If we are going to transform ourselves and society, it is only we as disabled people who can do the necessary intellectual work' and has criticised a range of disabled political activists from the Italian Marxist Antonio Gramsci to New Labour's Education Secretary David Blunkett for failing to 'embrace their impairments as part of a politics of personal identity' – in Gramsci's case at least, for seeing class, rather than disability, as the central divide within capitalism (Oliver 1996: 14).

To what extent, then, do such identity politics offer a way forward for mental health service users? Several factors would suggest that they don't. First, while people with mental health problems do experience oppression in many aspects of their lives, that oppression differs in important respects from that experienced by, say, women or blacks. Both women's oppression and the oppression of black people are central to the functioning of capitalism. Women's oppression, for example, is rooted in the family and in the way in which women can serve as a cheaper section of the workforce. Racism has its roots in the experience of colonialism and slavery and in the way in which it can still be used by the ruling class as a tool to 'divide and rule' workers. By contrast, the relatively small number of people experiencing mental health problems at any one time and the often hidden and transient nature of such problems means that the oppression they experience is much less systematic and, from the point of view of the ruling class, much less significant as a tool to 'divide and rule'.

Second, while there has been a growth in user self-organization and confidence over the past decade, there are a number of factors which are likely to limit that growth. The basis for any movement of oppressed people is a willingness on the part of individuals who belong to that group to stand up and challenge existing portrayals of that group – to 'come out', in the language of the gay movement. Yet, as Barnes and Shardlow note, the difficulties of doing so for people with mental health problems may be of a qualitatively different order:

making one's identity as a user of services visible may not be easy because of the stigma attached to such a status. In the case of people whose shared identity centres around their use of mental health services there are particular problems associated not only with the status of service user, but with the fear of madness.

(Barnes and Shardlow 1996: 115)

A member of a mental health project in Ayr, Scotland expressed the problem in the following way:

I'm here because I've no confidence. You see other people, they say ' G. was a union man'. But when you're in the hospital, you depend on the staff to help you, you look up to them. So when it comes to shouting the odds, you've no self-confidence. You can't go out into the street and walk up and down with a placard and shout 'I'm daft – what are you going to do about it?' You've had no self-confidence in the first place – you hide away.

The disincentives for people with mental health problems to 'come out' as part of a users' movement are considerable and include the implications for employment, housing and social relationships discussed earlier. While it may be possible for those who are in particular occupations or who are employed within voluntary organizations in the mental health field to do so, in general, even within the so-called 'caring professions' such as statutory social work, an admission of a mental health problem is likely to lead to the individual being treated with suspicion (*Community Care*, 17 September 1998). Given that the majority of people with mental health problems are likely to be poor or working class, the attractions of being a movement activist are likely to be limited. The comments of one writer regarding the difficulties of 'coming out' for working-class gays and lesbians seem apposite:

Obviously in a society where normalised heterosexuality and the family are pushed as the only valid expression of sexuality, individual 'coming out' is more or less the only way to reject dominant values and live as an out gay person. However, the vast majority of working-class people who experience lesbian or gay feelings cannot go through this individualised process because they do not have the necessary levels of independence, support and confidence to do so.

(Field 1995: 37–8)

There is another parallel with the position of gays which may inhibit involvement in a users' movement. While sexism, racism and disablism are usually forms of oppression based upon visible, physical characteristics, many mental health problems, such as depression or eating disorders or milder forms of schizophrenia, can be concealed or controlled through medication. Given the high costs of 'coming out', many may prefer to keep their mental health problems hidden – especially since, again unlike these other forms of oppression, they may be intermittent in nature.

Fourth, there is the impact of mental health problems in themselves and the implications of these problems for sustaining and developing collective organization. As one activist within the main Scottish users' organization, Scottish Users' Network, put it:

> We face all the usual pressures that apply to any organization but with an extra layer – our own mental health problems. The pressures mean that feelings can be more difficult to handle – that can create instability.

Fifth, as the earlier discussions on terminology and identity indicate, 'claiming' a mental health identity may not be the same as claiming a gay or a black identity. For many people, having a mental health problem is likely to be something they want to leave behind; while the spirit of 'glad to be mad' is a proud and defiant retort to the ignorance of stigma and discrimination, it was not a sentiment shared by the majority of the participants in the Scottish study referred to above. There, what respondents often valued most about the projects they attended was precisely that these projects did *not* focus on mental ill-health.

Finally, whatever common experiences users of mental health services may share, a politics of identity based on that experience which fails to recognize the centrality of the class divisions among service users discussed earlier can lead users' groups to claim some very strange bedfellows indeed. Thus, in late 1998 the magazine *Community Care* reported a demonstration involving several users' organizations against the Royal College of Psychiatrists' (RCP) launch of a 'Challenging Stigma' campaign (*Community Care*, 29 October 1998). With some justification, these groups were criticizing what they saw as the hypocrisy of the RCP campaign on the basis that individual psychiatrists and psychiatry as a profession had played a major role in both creating and sustaining this stigma over the decades. What was significant about this demonstration, however, was that, as the photograph accompanying the report showed, it took place beneath a statue of Sir Winston Churchill, the rationale being that as Churchill was a well-known sufferer from depression, he therefore shared a common interest with these service users. Leaving aside Churchill's well-documented attitude towards oppressed groups in general (including *inter alia* his ministerial involvement in the shooting down of striking Welsh miners in 1911 and his public admiration throughout the 1930s for Mussolini's fascists), as Clive Ponting has revealed in his biography of Churchill, he was also throughout his life a convinced eugenicist who, while a member of the 1906–14 Liberal government, went so far as to advocate the compulsory sterilisation of 100,000 of the 'mentally enfeebled' and the herding of many more into concentration camps as a basis for protecting the purity of the British 'race' (Ponting 1994). While the example may be an extreme one, it does serve to make the point that class interests will often be a far more potent basis for a shared identity than the experience of mental ill-health.

Marxism and oppression

Given the issues involved in developing a users' movement, it is perhaps not surprising that the importance of 'allies' is a frequent theme in the user literature. In discussing this issue, Mike Lawson, a leading member of the British users' movement, has written that:

> The collaboration between recipients and some workers in the UK is unique. There is no doubt that workers have helped the self-advocacy movement in this country to establish and continue to work in all kinds of settings. It is obvious that where we can work together we should.
>
> (Lawson 1991: 74)

As this statement suggests, 'allies' has tended to mean mental health workers (or occasionally, other disabled groups) while the relationship between users and allies is one of allies *supporting* user activities and initiatives. While such a position is preferable to the separatist stance of some sections of the American movement (Chamberlin 1988), it still raises issues of what kind of alliances are necessary if users are to successfully challenge their oppression and also what the relationship should be between users and allies. In this final section, I wish to sketch out an approach based on Marxism rather than identity politics, as the most effective way of addressing these issues.

The notion that Marxism is incapable of accounting for oppression and the movements that arise to challenge that oppression is at the heart of new social movement theory:

NSM theory developed partly in response to what was considered an outmoded style of class analysis ... the theory presumes that class analysis can no longer trace the main contours of social reality.

(Foweraker 1995: 36)

As we have seen, however, NSM theory's emphasis on identity and the identity politics to which that emphasis gives rise hardly provide a basis on which to challenge the oppression that users experience. By contrast, the classical Marxist tradition does suggest ways in which that oppression can be overcome.

In the context of the present discussion, three elements of that tradition are of particular significance. First, there is the central role of the working class as the agent of a socialist transformation of society. Space does not allow for a full discussion here of the thesis that the working class has disappeared or is no longer capable of acting as an agent of socialist change (Callinicos and Harman 1987; Ferguson and Lavalette 1999). Suffice it to say that not only is it the case that on a *world* scale the working class – including the industrial working class – has grown enormously over the past twenty-five years, but also within Britain and the rest of Europe, there are now millions of workers, including teachers, nurses and social workers, who two decades ago would not have seen themselves as working class and whose conditions of work bear more and more resemblance to those of manual workers. Since, for Marx, the working class is the only class in society capable of overthrowing the ruling class and beginning to build a society based on need and not profit, anything which weakens or creates divisions within that class must be opposed. Given that many varieties of oppression are employed to divide workers – straight against gay, white against black, or in this case, 'normal' versus 'mad' or 'loony' – combating that oppression is in the interests of *all* workers, not just those who experience the particular form of oppression. In the classic statement by Lenin of this position:

Working-class consciousness cannot be genuine political con-sciousness unless the workers are trained to respond to *all* cases of tyranny, oppressions, violence and abuse, no matter *what class* is affected – unless they are trained to respond from a Social Democratic [i.e. revolutionary socialist] point of view and no other.

(Lenin 1967 [1902]: 412)

In the case of the oppression of people with mental health problems, such a response is not based on a vague altruism but rather on a recognition that the vast majority of ordinary people suffer from such oppression. With one in seven people likely to experience mental health problems at some time in their lives (Metzer *et al.* 1994) and stress identified by 6,000 health and safety representatives in a Trades Union Congress (TUC) survey as the single major health and safety issue experienced by workers (TUC 1998), stigmatizing people with mental health problems creates a climate in which people are afraid to seek help, while the structural roots of these problems within the capitalist family and work process are obscured and unchallenged, removing the possibility of a collective response.

The second strand of the Marxist analysis of oppression is that not only does the working class have an *interest* in challenging all forms of oppression but it is also the only social force that has the *power* to do so. This power stems from its position within the process of production and the collective organization to which that gives rise. Members of oppressed groups by contrast tend to be more fragmented and isolated. Their lack of power can lead them to seek more powerful allies, which in the British context has often meant looking towards a Labour government.

Significantly, Rogers and Pilgrim, who have been among the main proponents of NSM theory in respect of service users, writing shortly before the election of New Labour, hinted at precisely such a strategy when they wrote that:

> it may be that old and new social movements are being brought together rather than being separated. What is currently missing in regard to the influence of the mental health users' movements is the opportunity of a Labour government to be tested in its commitment in practice to a new pluralistic health and welfare agenda.
>
> (Rogers and Pilgrim 1996: 171)

In fact, two years after the election of a New Labour government in 1997, it was clear that, if anything, that government was going further than its predecessor in its emphasis on 'dangerousness', with the then Health Minister, for example, seriously considering the introduction of compulsory measures of treatment in the community – a measure abandoned by the Conservatives in the face of fierce opposition from a wide range of bodies including MIND and the British Association of Social Workers (*OpenMind*, November/December 1998; *Guardian*, 9 December 1988). While a range of new mental health services, including 24-hour crisis centres, has also been promised, the government's emphasis on fiscal rectitude on the one hand and its repeated insistence that 'community care has failed' on the other, suggest that the emphasis will still be on controlling behaviour rather than developing the range of community-based services which users and mental health workers have been campaigning for (Clements 1998).

Against this, it might be argued that there are few examples of mental health users' groups seeking to form alliances with trade unionists. Barnes and Shardlow, for example, suggest that 'there is little evidence of groups allying themselves with class based movements' (1996: 127). As I have argued elsewhere, however, such alliances can be built (Ferguson 1999). As was mentioned above, several Scottish users' groups including the Scottish Users' Network, the Edinburgh Users' Forum and Saheliya, a project for minority ethnic women with mental health problems, supported a national demonstration called by the Scottish Trades Union Congress in early 1997 against cuts in local authority funding. What this suggests is that the lack of evidence for alliances of users' and class-based movements is a contingent rather than a necessary or essential feature of the users' movement.

Finally, the recognition that, as argued above, the majority of working-class people suffer from the stigmatizing of mental ill-health and therefore share an interest in challenging that stigma, suggests a different kind of relationship between service users and other socialists and activists. On the one hand, it suggests a need within the trade union movement to challenge the stigma surrounding mental ill-health, in the same way as other forms of discrimination and oppression such as racism, sexism and homophobia have been challenged in recent years. On the other, it suggests that rather than the task of 'allies' of the users' movement being to uncritically support whatever initiatives or activities users are involved in – as though there were no political differences amongst users themselves – a relationship of mutual respect needs to be developed, based on debate and discussion of the best way forward for all those involved in challenging the exploitation and oppression which capitalism creates.

Conclusion

A central theme of this volume is the way in which popular struggles from below can challenge and shape welfare policies. Until very recently, users of mental health services have, along with disabled people and elderly people, been very much the objects rather than the subjects of such policies. The growth of a mental health users' movement over the past decade has begun to challenge that situation as far as people with mental health problems are concerned. If the challenge is to be sustained, however, it will have to overcome two main dangers.

First, there is the danger of service users and their organizations being sucked into endless 'consultations' or given responsibility for managing community-based services under the rhetoric of 'empowerment', at a time when both government and local authorities are withdrawing from the provision of welfare services. While the attractions of such involvement are obvious for people who have traditionally been denied any say over the services they receive, the dangers in the situation were succinctly summed up by a leading Scottish activist at the Scottish Users' Conference mentioned earlier:

> There's been a sea-change in attitudes in the past few years. People have been going overboard to involve us in consultation – the Scottish Office, the Health Board and so on. My cynicism may be proved wrong but while we're talking about making improvements, the powers that be have been making cuts. ... Without money to back up services, it's just a talking shop. We will not sit passively by and watch our lives being destroyed by intolerable funding cuts. Don't give us something and then take it away again. To take funds away from a project that is working is obscene.

Second, there is the danger that in the face of increased scapegoating by both media and government, there will be an increase in the influence of an identity politics within the users' movement which sees 'non-users' as 'the enemy', leading to greater internalization. Yet the experience of the 1997 campaign in Scotland against cuts in community-based services suggests that it is when service users make common cause with public sector trade unionists and other groups in defence of services that they are most effective. Nor should this surprise us. For as other chapters in this book illustrate, it is precisely at such high points in the struggle, when the anger of oppressed groups is fused with the collective power of organized workers, that the possibility for overcoming racist or sexist or stigmatizing ideas regarding mental ill-health is at its greatest, as is the potential for challenging a system which systematically oppresses and denigrates those who fail to meet its requirements for participation in the market.

Bibliography

Adler, A. (ed.) (1980) *Theses, Resolutions and Manifestos of the First Four Congresses of the Third International*, London: Ink Links.

Anderson, P. (1976) *Considerations on Western Marxism*, London: NLB.

Anning, N., Wates, N. and Woolmar, C. (eds) (1980) *Squatting: The Real Story*, London: Bayleaf Books.

Arnold, A. (1888) 'Socialism and the unemployed', *Contemporary Review*, 53: 560–71.

Aronowitz, S. (1992) *The Politics of Identity: Class, Culture, Social Movements*, London: Routledge.

Atherley-Jones, L. (1893) 'Liberalism and social reform: A warning', *The New Review* 9: 629–35.

Aya, R. (1979) 'Theories of revolution reconsidered: Contrasting models of collective violence', *Theory and Society* 8(1): 39–99.

Baggley, P. (1996) 'The moral economy of the poll tax', in C. Barker and P. Kennedy (eds), *To Make Another World: Studies in Protest and Collective Action*, Aldershot: Ashgate.

Bagguley, P. and Mann, K. (1992) 'Idle, thieving bastards: Scholarly representations of the underclass', *Work, Employment and Society* 6(1): 113–26.

Barham, P. and Hayward, R. (1995) *Relocating Madness: From the Mental Patient to the Person*, London: Free Association Press.

Barker, C. and Dale, G. (1999), 'Protest waves in Western Europe: A critique of "new social movement" theory', *Critical Sociology* 24(1/2): 65–104.

Barker, C., Johnson, A. and Lavalette, M. (eds) (forthcoming a) *Leadership and Social Movements*, Manchester: Manchester University Press.

—— (eds) (forthcoming b) *Constructing Strategies, Transforming Identities*, Liverpool: Liverpool University Press.

Barker, C. and Kennedy, P. (eds) (1996) *To Make Another World: Studies in Protest and Collective Action*, Aldershot: Ashgate.

Barker, M. (1981) *The New Racism: Conservatives and the Ideology of the Tribe*, London: Junction Books.

Barker, M. and Beezer, A. (1983) 'The language of racism – an examination of Lord Scarman's Report on the Brixton riots', *International Socialism* 18: 108–25.

Barnes, M. (1997) *Care, Communities and Citizens*, London: Longman.

Barnes, M. and Shardlow, P. (1996) 'Identity crisis: mental health user groups and the "problem" of identity', in C. Barnes and G. Mercer, *Exploring the Divide: Illness and Disability*, Leeds: The Disability Press.

Barton, L. (ed.) (1996) *Disability and Society: Emerging Issues and Insights*, London: Longman.

Beier, A. L. (1983) *The Problem of the Poor in Tudor and Early Stuart England*, London: Methuen.

Benhabib, S. (1995) 'From identity politics to social feminism: A plea for the nineties', in D. Trend (ed.), *Radical Democracy: Identity, Citizenship and the State*, New York: Routledge.

Benson, J. (1975) 'English coal-miners' trade-union accident funds, 1850–1900', *Economic History Review* XXVIII(3): 401–12.

Benyon, J. (ed.) (1984) *Scarman and After*, Oxford: Pergamon Press.

Benyon, J. and Solomos, J. (1987) 'British urban unrest in the 1980s', in J. Benyon and J. Solomos (eds), *The Roots of Urban Unrest*, Oxford: Pergamon Press.

Berer, M. (1988) 'Whatever happened to a woman's right to choose?', *Feminist Review* 29, Spring: 24–37.

Bhavnani, R., Coke, J., Gilroy, P., Hall, S., Ouseley, H. and Vaz, K. (1986) *Different Reality: An Account of Black People's Experiences and their Grievances Before and After the Handsworth Rebellions of September 1985*, Report of the Review Panel, West Midlands County Council.

Binion, G. (1991) 'Webster v. Reproductive Health Services: devaluing the right to choose', *Women and Politics* 11(2): 41–59.

Blair, T. (1998) *The Third Way*, London: Fabian Society.

Blakemore, K. (1998) *Social Policy: An Introduction*, Buckingham: Open University Press.

Boddy, M. and Fudge, C. (eds) (1984) *Local Socialism?*, London: Macmillan.

Bonner, A. (1961) *British Co-operation: The History, Principles, and Organisation of the British Co-operative Movement*, Manchester: Co-operative Union.

Booth, C. (1889) *Life and Labour of the People, Volume 1*, London: Macmillan.

Boyle, M. (1991) *Schizophrenia: A Scientific Delusion*, London: Routledge.

The Bradford Commission (1996) *The Report of an Inquiry into the Wider Implications of Public Disorders in Bradford which Occurred in Bradford on 9, 10, and 11 June 1995*, London: The Stationery Office.

Branson, N. (1975) *Britain in the Nineteen Twenties*, London: Weidenfeld and Nicholson.

—— (1979) *Poplarism 1919–1925. George Lansbury and the Councillors' Revolt*, London: Lawrence and Wishart.

Branson, N. and Heinemann, M. (1973) *Britain in the Nineteen Thirties*, London: Panther.

Breggin, P. (1993) *Toxic Psychiatry*, London: Harper Collins.

Breggin, P. and Breggin, G. (1995) *Talking Back to Prozac*, New York: St Martin's Press.

Brenner, J. (1993) 'The best of times, the worst of times: US feminism today', *New Left Review* 200, July/August: 100–59.

Briggs, A. and Saville, J. (eds) (1960) *Essays in Labour History*, London: Methuen.

Brogan, C. (1952) *The Glasgow Story*, London: Fredrick Muller.

Brookes, B. (1988) *Abortion in England 1960–1967*, London: Croom Helm.

Brown, G. and Harris, T. (1978) *Social Origins of Depression: A Study of Psychiatric Disorder in Women*, London: Tavistock.

Brown, R. (1991) *Abortion – A Woman's Right to Choose*, London: Socialist Workers Party.

Brown, R. and Daniels, C. (1984) *The Chartists*, London: Macmillan.

Bruce, M. (1968) *The Coming of the Welfare State* (4th edn.), London: Batsford.

Bryher, S. (1929) 'Labour and socialist movement in Bristol', *Bristol Labour Weekly*, June.

Bunyan, T. (1981–2) 'The police against the people', *Race and Class* XXIII(2/3): 153–70.

Burns, D. (1992) *Poll Tax Rebellion*, Stirling: AK Press.

Busfield, J. (1986) *Managing Madness*, London: Hutchinson.

—— (1996) *Men, Women and Madness: Understanding Gender and Mental Disorder*, Basingstoke: Macmillan.

Butler, D., Adonis, A. and Travers, T. (1994) *Failure in British Government: The Politics of the Poll Tax*, Oxford: Oxford University Press.

Butt, J. (1978) 'Working-class housing in Glasgow, 1900–1939', in I. MacDougall (ed.), *Essays in Scottish Labour History*, Edinburgh: John Donald.

—— (1987) 'Housing', in R. A. Cage (ed.), *The Working Class in Glasgow, 1750–1914*, London: Croom Helm.

Byrne, D. (1982) 'Class and the local state', *International Journal of Urban and Regional Research* 6(1): 61–82.

Calder, A. (1969) *The People's War*, London: Cape.

Callinicos, A. (1989) *Against PostModernism*, Cambridge: Polity.

—— (1993) *Race and Class*, London: Bookmarks.

—— (1995) *Theories and Narratives*, Cambridge: Polity.

—— (1999) *Social Theory*, Cambridge: Polity.

Callinicos, A. and Harman, C. (1987) *The Changing Working Class*, London: Bookmarks.

Callinicos, A. and Simons, M. (1985) *The Great Strike*, London: Socialist Workers Party.

Campbell, B. (1993) *Goliath: Britain's Dangerous Places*, London: Methuen.

Campbell, P. (1996) 'The history of the user movement in the United Kingdom', in T. Heller, J. Reynolds, R. Gomm, R. Muston and S. Pattison, *Mental Health Matters: A Reader*, Basingstoke: Macmillan.

Castells, M. (1983) *The City and the Grassroots*, London: Edward Arnold.

Chamberlain, J. (1892) 'Old age pensions and friendly societies', *The National Review* (24): 592–615.

Chamberlin, J. (1988) *On Our Own*, London: MIND.

Charlesworth, A., Gilbert, D., Randall, A. and Southall, H. (1996), *An Atlas of Industrial Life in Britain: 1750–1990*, Basingstoke: Macmillan.

Charlton, J. (1992) 'Working Class Structure and Working Class Politics in Britain 1750–1939', unpublished Ph.D. thesis, University of Leeds.

—— (1999) *'It All Went Like Tinder': The Rise and Fall of a Mass Movement*, London: Redwords.

Clegg, S. (1996) 'From the women's movement to feminism', in C. Barker and P. Kennedy (eds), *To Make Another World: Studies in Protest and Collective Action*, Aldershot: Ashgate.

Clements, J. (1998) 'A Third Way for mental illness?', *Community Care*, 10–16 December: 16–22.

Cliff, T. (1957) 'Economic roots of reformism', in T. Cliff (1982) *Neither Washington Nor Moscow: Essays in Revolutionary Socialism*, London: Bookmarks.

Cliff, T. and Gluckstein, D. (1988) *The Labour Party: A Marxist Analysis*, London: Bookmarks.

Cohan, A. (1986) 'Abortion as a marginal issue: The use of peripheral mechanism in Britain and the United States', in J. Lovenduski and J. Outshoorn (eds), *The New Politics of Abortion*, London: Sage.

Collins, C. (1996) 'To concede or to contest? Language and the class struggle', in C. Barker and P. Kennedy (eds.), *To Make Another World: Studies in Protest and Collective Action*, Aldershot: Ashgate.

Committee on the Rent Restrictions Act (1925) *Report of the Committee on the Rent Restriction Act*, Cmd., 2423, 1925 (the 'Constable Commission').

Committee on the 1920 Rent Restrictions Act (1923) *Report of the Committee on the 1920 Rent Restriction Act*, Cmd., 1803, 1923 (the 'Onslow Committee').

Confidential Inquiry 1994 (1994) *A Preliminary Report on Homicide*, London: Steering Committee.

Corrigan, Paul (1979) *Schooling the Smash St Kids*, London: Macmillan.

Corrigan, Philip (1977) 'State formation and moral regulation in nineteenth century Britain', unpublished Ph.D. thesis, University of Durham.

Cowell, D., Jones, T. and Young, J. (1982) *Policing the Riots*, London: Junction Books.

Cowherd, R. G. (1977) *Economists and the English Poor Laws*, Ohio: Ohio University Press.

Coyle, A. (1988) 'Continuity and change: Women in paid work', in A. Coyle and J. Skinner (eds), *Women and Work: Positive Action for Change*, Hampshire: Macmillan.

Crawfurd, H. (n.d.) *Autobiography*, typescript MSS in the Marx Memorial Library, London.

Crepaz-Keay, D. (1996) 'A sense of perspective: The media and the Boyd Inquiry', in G. Philo (ed.), *Media and Mental Distress*, London: Longman.

Croucher, R. (1987) *We Refuse to Starve in Silence: A History of the National Unemployed Workers Movement*, London: Lawrence and Wishart.

Cunningham, H. (1980) *Leisure in the Industrial Revolution*, London: Croom Helm.

Damer, S. (1980) 'Housing, class and state', in J. Melling (ed.), *Housing, State and Social Policy*, London: Croom Helm.

—— (1982) *Rent Strike! The Clydebank Rent Struggles of the 1920s*, Clydebank: Clydebank District Libraries People's History Pamphlet.

—— (1985) 'State, local state and local struggle: The Clydebank Rent Strike of the 1920s', Glasgow University, CURR Discussion Paper no. 22.

—— (1990) *Glasgow: Going For a Song*, London: Lawrence and Wishart.

Davies, A. (1982) *Women, Race and Class*, London: Women's Press.

Davin, A. (1978) 'Imperialism and motherhood', *History Workshop* 5, Spring: 9–65.

—— (1996) *Growing Up Poor: Home, School and Street in London, 1870–1914*, London: Riversoram.

Davis, M. (1992), 'The rebellion that rocked a superpower', *Socialist Review*, June: 8–11.

—— (1993a) 'Who killed LA? A political autopsy', *New Left Review* 197.

—— (1993b) 'Who killed LA? Part 2: The verdict is given', *New Left Review* 199.

De Ste Croix, G. (1981) *The Class Struggle in the Ancient Greek World*, London: Ducksworth.

Deakin, N. (1994) *The Politics of Welfare: Continuities and Change*, London: Harvester Wheatsheaf.

Dear, G. (1985) *Report of the Chief Constable, West Midlands Police, on Handsworth/Lozells Disturbances*, September 1985, Birmingham: West Midlands Police.

Department of the Environment (1994) 'Assessing the impact of urban policy', *Inner Cities Research Programme*, London: HMSO.

Derrida, J. (1994) *The Spectre of Marx*, London: Routledge.

Digby, A. (1982) *The Poor Law in Nineteenth Century England and Wales*, London: The History Association.

Digby, F. (1978) *Pauper Palaces*, London, RKP.

Dobson, R. B. (1983) *The Peasants Revolt of 1381*, Basingstoke: Macmillan.

Donaldson, N. and Forster, L. (1993) *Sell and Be Damned: The Glasgow Merrylee Scandal of 1951* (unpublished).

Draper, H. (1996) *The Two Souls of Socialism* (1st edn. 1966), London: Bookmarks.

Driver, S. and Martell, L. (1998) *New Labour: Politics After Thatcherism*, Cambridge: Polity.

Eagleton, T. (1996) *The Illusions of Postmodernism*, Oxford: Blackwell.

Edsall, N. C. (1971) *The Anti-Poor Law Movement*, Manchester: Manchester University Press.

Ehrenreich, B. and English, D. (1979) *For Her Own Good: 150 Years of the Experts' Advice to Women*, London: Pluto Press.

Ellison, N. (1998) 'The changing politics of social policy', in N. Ellison and C. Pierson (eds), *Developments in British Social Policy*, London: Macmillan.

Ellison, N. and Pierson, C. (eds) (1998) *Developments in British Social Policy*, London: Macmillan.

Engels, F. (1958) *The Condition of the Working Class in England*, Oxford: Blackwell.

—— (1962 [1892]) 'Preface' to the English edition (1892) of 'The condition of the working class in England', in K. Marx and F. Engels, *On Britain*, Moscow: Progress.

Englander, D. (1983) *Landlord and Tenant in Urban Britain 1838–1918*, Oxford: Oxford University Press.

Esping-Anderson, G. (1990) *The Three Worlds of Welfare Capitalism*, Oxford: Polity.

Farrell, A. (1992) *Crime, Class and Corruption*, London: Bookmarks.

Ferguson, I. (1999) 'The potential and limits of mental health service user involvement', unpublished Ph.D. thesis, University of Glasgow.

Ferguson, I. and Lavalette, M. (1999) 'Postmodernism, Marxism and social work', *European Journal of Social Work* 2(1): 27–40.

Fernando, S. (ed.) (1995) *Mental Health in a Multi-ethnic Society*, London: Routledge.

Fied, M. G. (1998) 'Abortion in the United States – legal but inaccessible', in R. Solinger (ed.), *Abortion Wars – A Half Century of Struggle 1950–2000*, California: University of California Press.

Field, N. (1995) *Over the Rainbow: Money, Class and Homophobia*, London: Pluto Press.

Fishman, W. L. (1975) *East End Jewish Radicals 1875–1914*, London: Duckworth.

Foot, M. (1975) *Aneurin Bevan, 1945–1960*, Herts: Paladin.

Foot, P. (1965) *Immigration and Race in British Politics*, Harmondsworth: Penguin Books.

Foster, J. (1979) 'How imperial London preserved its slums', *International Journal of Urban and Regional Research* 3(1): 93–114.

Foweraker, J. (1995) *Theorizing Social Movements*, London: Pluto Press.

Fox-Piven, F. and Cloward, R. A. (1977) *Poor People's Movements: Why They Succeed, How They Fail*, New York: Pantheon Books.

Francome, C. (1986) *Abortion Practice in Britain and the United States*, London: Allen and Unwin.

Fraser, D. (1973) *The Evolution of the British Welfare State*, London: Macmillan.

—— (1984) *The Evolution of the British Welfare State* (2nd edn.), London: Macmillan.

Friedan, B. (1965) *The Feminine Mystique*, London: Penguin.

Gaffney, J. (1987) 'Interpretations of violence: the Handsworth riots of 1985', *Policy Papers in Ethnic Relations, no. 10*, University of Warwick.

Gallagher, W. (1978) *Revolt on the Clyde*, London: Lawrence and Wishart.

George, V. and Miller, S. (eds) (1994) *Social Policy: Towards 2000*, London: Routledge.

Geras, N. (1990) *Discourses of Extremity. Radical Ethics and Post-Modern Extravagances*, London: Verso.

Geremek, B. (1997) *Poverty: A History*, Oxford: Blackwell.

German, L. (1988) 'The rise and fall of the women's movement', *International Socialism*, 2(37): 3–47.

German, L. (1989) *Sex, Class and Socialism*, London: Bookmarks.

—— (1990) 'The last days of Thatcher?', *International Socialism* 48.

Gibb, A. (1983) *Glasgow: The Making of a City*, London: Croom Helm.

Gilbert, B. (1964) 'The decay of nineteenth century provident institutions and the coming of old age pensions in Great Britain', *Economic History Review* XVII(3): 551–63.

—— (1966) *The Evolution of National Insurance in Great Britain: The Origins of the Welfare State*, London: Michael Joseph.

Gilroy, P. (1981/2) 'You can't fool the youths', *Race and Class*, XXIII(2/3): 207–22.

—— (1987) *There Ain't No Black in the Union Jack*, London: Unwin Hyman.

Ginsburg, N. (1979) *Class, Capital and Social Policy*, London: Macmillan.

—— (1992) *Divisions of Welfare*, London: Sage.

Gitlin, T. (1994) 'The rise of "identity politics" ', in N. Mills (ed.), *Legacy of Dissent. 40 Years of Writing from Dissent Magazine*, New York: Simon and Schuster.

Glasgow Corporation (1943) *Annual Report of the Medical Officer of Health*, Glasgow: Glasgow Corporation.

Goffman, E. (1961) *Asylums*, Harmondsworth: Penguin.

Gomm, R. (1996) 'Mental health and inequality', in T. Heller, J. Reynolds, R. Gomm, R. Muston and S. Pattison (eds), *Mental Health Matters: A Reader*, Basingstoke: Macmillan.

Goodwin, S. (1990) *Community Care and the Future of Mental Health Service Provision*, Aldershot: Avebury.

Gough, I. (1979) *The Political Economy of the Welfare State*, London: Macmillan.

Gramsci, A. (1971) *Selections From the Prison Notebooks*, London: Lawrence and Wishart.

Graves, P. M. (1994) *Labour Women – Women in British Working Class Politics 1918–1939*, Cambridge: University of Cambridge Press.

Gray, N. (ed.) (1985) *The Worst of Times*, London: Wildwood House.

Greater London Council (GLC) (1985) *London Industrial Strategy*, London: GLC.

Greenwood, V. and Young, J. (1976) *Abortion in Demand*, London: Pluto Press.

Hall, S. and Jacques, M. (1989) *New Times*, London: Lawrence and Wishart.

Hammond, J. L. and Hammond, B. (1995 [1925]) *The Town Labourer: The New Civilisation, 1760–1832*, London: Alan Sutton/Longmans.

Harman, C. (1981) 'The summer of 1981: A post-riot analysis', *International Socialism* 14: 1–43.

—— (1985) '1984 and the shape of things to come', *International Socialism* 29: 62–127.

Heclo, H. (1974) *Modern Social Politics in Britain and Sweden*, New Haven: Yale University Press.

Heller, T., Reynolds, J., Gomm, R., Muston, R. and Pattison, S. (eds) (1996) *Mental Health Matters: A Reader*, Basingstoke: Macmillan.

Henderson, C., Thornicroft, G. and Glover, G. (1998) 'Inequalities in mental health', *British Journal of Psychiatry* 173: 105–9.

Hendrick, H. (1974) 'The Leeds gas strike 1890', Thoresby Society: Miscellany.

Hill, C. (1993) *The Century of Revolution 1603–1714*, London: Routledge.

—— (1994) *Puritanism and Revolution*, London: Secker and Warburg.

Hill, M. (1993) *The Welfare State in Britain*, Aldershot: Edward Elgar.

Hills, J. (1996) 'Introduction: After the turning point', in J. Hills (ed.), *New Inequalities: The Changing Distribution of Income and Wealth in the United Kingdom*, Cambridge: Cambridge University Press.

Hindell, K. and Simms, M. (1968) 'How the abortion lobby worked', *Political Quarterly* 39: 269–82.

—— (1977) *Abortion Law Reformed*, London: Peter Owen.

Hobsbawm, E. J. (1978) *Industry and Empire*, Harmondsworth: Penguin.

—— (1984) 'The making of the working class 1870–1914', in *Worlds of Labour*, London: Nicholson.

—— (1987) *Age of Empire: 1875–1914*, London: Abacus.

Hogg, Q. (1944) *Parliamentary Proceedings, Volume 386* Col. 1918.

Hoggart, R. (1960) 'The welfare state: Appearance and reality', *Social Work* 17: 13–17.

Hoggett, P. and Burns, D. (1991) 'The revenge of the poor: The anti-poll tax campaign in Britain', *Critical Social Policy* 33: 95–110.

Hollis, P. (1973) *Class and Conflict in Nineteenth Century England 1815–1850*, London: Routledge and Kegan Paul.

Holyoake, G. (1878) 'The new principle of industry', *Nineteenth Century* 4: 494–511.

Home Office (1992) *Criminal Statistics England and Wales 1990* Cmnd. 1935, London: HMSO.

—— (1997) *Criminal Statistics England and Wales 1996*, Cmnd. 3764, London: HMSO.

Hood, J. (ed.) (1988) *The History of Clydebank*, Lancs: Carnforth.

Hopkins, E. (1979) *A Social History of the English Working Classes*, London: Hodder and Stoughton.

Hughes, G. and Lewis, G. (eds) (1998) *Unsettling Welfare*, London: Routledge.

Inglis, K. S. (1963) *Churches and the Working Classes in Victorian England*, London: Routledge and Kegan Paul.

Issac, J. (1994) 'The politics of morality in the UK', *Parliamentary Affairs* 47(2): 175–89.

Jewell, H. (1990) '*Piers Plowman* – a poem of crisis: An analysis of political instability in Langland's England', in C. Taylor and R. Childs (eds), *Politics and Crisis in Fourteenth Century England*, Gloucester: Wiley.

Johnson, A. (1996) 'Militant and the failure of "acherontic" Marxism in Liverpool', in C. Barker and P. Kennedy (eds), *To Make Another World: Studies in Protest and Collective Action*, Aldershot: Ashgate.

Johnson, A. (forthcoming) 'Equality with a difference: The campaign for a "Labor Equal Rights Amendment" in California', in C. Barker, A. Johnson and M. Lavalette (eds) *Constructing Strategies, Transforming Identities*, Liverpool: Liverpool University Press.

Johnson, N. (1990) *Reconstructing the Welfare State*, London: Harvester Wheatsheaf.

Jones, C. and Novak, T. (1985) 'Welfare against the workers: Benefits as a political weapon', in H. Beynon (ed.), *Digging Deeper*, London: Verso.

Jones, C. and Novak, T. (1999) *Poverty, Welfare and the Disciplinary State*, London: Routledge.

Jones, H. and MacGregor, S. (eds) (1998) *Social Issues and Party Politics*, London: Routledge.

Jones, K. (1991) *The Making of Social Policy in Britain 1830–1990*, London: The Athlone Press.

Judd, R. W. (1989) *Socialist Cities. Municipal Politics and the Grass Roots of American Socialism*, Albany: State University of New York Press.

Keith, M. (1993) *Race, Riots and Policing: Lore and Disorder in a Multi-racist Society*, London: UCL Press.

Kenefick, W. and McIvor, A. (1996) *The Roots of Red Clydeside 1910–1914*, Edinburgh: John Donald.

Kerner, O. (1968) *Report of the National Advisory Commission on Civil Disorders (The Kerner Report)*, New York: Bantam Books.

Kesselman, A. (1988) 'Woman v. Connecticut: Conducting a statewide hearing on abortion', in R. Solinger (ed.), *Abortion Wars – A Half Century of Struggle 1950–2000*, California: University of California Press.

Kettle, M. and Hodges, L. (1982) *Uprising!: The Police, the People and the Riots in Britain's Cities*, London: Pan Books.

Kingsford, P. (1982) *The Hunger Marches in Britain*, London: Lawrence and Wishart.

Klandermans, B. (1997) *The Social Psychology of Protest*, Oxford: Blackwell.

Knott, J. (1986) *Popular Opposition to the 1834 Poor Law*, London: Croom Helm.

Kotowicz, Z. (1997) *R. D. Laing and the Paths of Anti-Psychiatry*, London: Routledge.

Labour Briefing Scotland (1988) *Labour, the Assembly and the Poll Tax*, Glasgow: Labour Briefing Scotland.

Laclau, E. (ed.) (1994) *The Making of Political Identities*, London: Verso.

Laing, R. D. (1964) *The Divided Self*, Harmondsworth: Penguin Books.

Langan, M. and Schwarz, B. (eds) (1985) *Crisis in the British State*, London: Hutchinson.

Lansbury, E. (1933) *George Lansbury, My Father*, London: Sampson Low, Marston and Co.

Lansbury, G. (1928) *My Life*, London: Constable and Co.

Larkin, M. (1994) *£500 Million More*, Surrey: NSF.

Laski, H. (1928) 'Introduction', in G. Lansbury, *My Life*, London: Constable and Co.

Lavalette, M. (1994) *Child Employment in the Capitalist Labour Market*, Aldershot: Ashgate.

—— (1997) 'Marx and Marxist critique of welfare', in M. Lavalette and A. Pratt, *Social Policy: Conceptual and Theoretical Introduction*, London: Sage.

Lavalette, M. and Kennedy, J. (1996) *Solidarity on the Waterfront: The First Year of the Liverpool Lock-Out*, Liverpool: Liver Press.

Lavalette, M. and Mooney, G. (1989) 'The struggle against the poll tax in Scotland', *Critical Social Policy* 26: 82–100.

—— (1990) 'Undermining the North–South divide? Fighting the poll tax in Scotland, England and Wales', *Critical Social Policy* 29: 100–19.

—— (1992/93) 'The poll tax struggle in Britain: A reply to Hoggett and Burns', *Critical Social Policy* 36: 96–108.

Lavalette, M. and Pratt, A. (1996) *Social Policy: A Conceptual and Theoretical Introduction*, London: Sage.

Lawson, M. (1991) 'A recipient's view', in S. Ramon (ed.), *Beyond Community Care*, London: Macmillan.

Le Bon, G. (1903) *The Crowd: A Study of the Popular Mind*, London: T. Fisher Unwin.

Le Grand, J. (1990) *Quasi-Markets and Social Policy*, Bristol: SAUS.

Lea, J. and Young, J. (1982) 'The riots in Britain 1981: Urban violence and political marginalisation', in D. Cowell, T. Jones and J. Young, *Policing the Riots*, London: Junction Books.

Lenin, V. I. (1977 [1920]) 'Left wing communism: An infantile disorder', in *Selected Works Volume 3*, Moscow: Progress Publishers.

—— (1967 [1902]) 'What is to be done?', in *Collected Works Volume 5*, Moscow: Progress Publishers.

Lewis, G. (ed.) (1998) *Forming Nation, Framing Welfare*, London: Routledge.

Lindow, V. (1995) 'Power and rights: The psychiatric system survivor movement', in R. Jack (ed.), *Empowerment in Community Care*, London: Chapman and Hall.

Lister, R. (1998) *The Inclusive Society*, London: Macmillan.

Littlewood, R. and Lipsedge, M. (1989) *Aliens and Alienists: Ethnic Minorities and Psychiatry* (2nd edn.), London: Unwin Hyman.

Local Government Board for Scotland (1918) (LGBS) *Women's Housing Report*, LGBS.

Ludlam, S. and Smith, M. J. (eds) (1996) *Contemporary British Conservatism*, Basingstoke: Macmillan.

McCarthy, M. (1989) *The New Politics of Welfare*, London: Macmillan.

McConnell, A. (1989) 'The birth of the poll tax', *Critical Social Policy* 28: 67–78.

McLaren, A. (1978) *Birth Control in Nineteenth Century England*, London: Croom Helm.

McLean, I. (1983) *The Legend of Red Clydeside*, Edinburgh: John Donald.

MacLeod, R. (1983) 'The road to full employment', in H. Smith, *War and Social Change*, Manchester: Manchester University Press.

McShane, H. and Smith, J. (1978) *No Mean Fighter*, London: Pluto Press.

Mahon, J. (1978) *Harry Pollitt: A Biography*, London: Lawrence and Wishart.

Manning, B. (1996) *Aristocrats, Plebeians and Revolution in England 1640–1660*, London: Pluto Press.

Marquand, D. (1977) *Ramsay MacDonald*, London: Cape.

—— (1987) *The Unprincipled Society*, London: Fontana.

Marshall, J. D. (1968) *The Old Poor Law*, London: Macmillan.

Marx, K. (1969 [1875]) *Selected Works Volume 3,* Moscow: Progress Publishers.

—— (1971 [1847]) *The Poverty of Philosophy*, London: Lawrence and Wishart.

—— (1973 [1848]) 'Manifesto of the Communist Party', in D. Fernbach (ed.), *The Revolutions of 1848. Political Writings, Volume 1*, London: Penguin.

—— (1988 [1867]) *Capital, Volume 1*, Harmondsworth: Penguin and NLR.

Mastboom, J. C. M. (1992) 'Forty clubhouses: Models and practices', *Psychosocial Rehabilitaion Journal* 16(2): 9–23.

Mastermann, C. F. G. (1960) *The Condition of England*, London: Methuen.

Meacham, S. (1977) *A Life Apart: The English Working Class 1890–1914*, London: Thames and Hudson.

Melling, J. (1980) *Housing, State and Social Policy*, London: Croom Helm.

—— (1983) *Rent Strikes: Peoples' Struggle for Housing in West Scotland 1890–1916*, Edinburgh: Polygon.

Melzer, H., Gill, B. and Petticrew, M. (1994) *The Prevalence of Psychiatric Morbidity Among Adults Age 16–64, Living in Private Households in Britain*, London: OPCS.

Merseyside Socialist Research Group (1992) *Genuinely Seeking Work*, Liverpool: Liver Press.

Middlemas, K. (1979) *Politics in Industrial Society*, London: Macmillan.

Midwinter, A. and Monaghan, C. (1993) *From Rates to the Poll Tax*, Edinburgh: Edinburgh University Press.

Miles, R. and Phizacklea, A. (1984) *White Man's Country*, London: Pluto Press.

Miliband, R. (1972) *Parliamentary Socialism: A Study in the Politics of Labour*, London: Merlin Press.

Milton, N. (1973) *John Maclean*, London: Pluto Press.

Mitchell, A. (1998) 'Advancing the inter-group dynamic model in a post-disorder environment', in C. Barker and M. Tyldsley (eds), *The Proceedings of the Fourth International Conference on Alternative Futures and Popular Protest*, 15–17 April 1998, Manchester: MMU.

Mooney, G. (1998) 'Remoralising the poor? Gender, class and philanthropy in Victorian Britain', in G. Lewis (ed.), *Forming Nation, Framing Welfare*, London: Routledge.

—— (2000) 'Class and social policy', in G. Lewis, S. Gerwitz, and J. Clarke (eds), *Rethinking Social Policy*, London: Sage.

Moorhouse, B., Wilson, M. and Chamberlain, C. (1972) 'Rent strikes: Direct action and the working class', in R. Miliband and J. Saville (eds), *The Socialist Register*, London: Merlin Press.

Morgan, K. (1993) *Harry Pollitt*, Manchester: Manchester University Press.

Nairn, T. (1972) 'The English working class', in R. Blackburn, *Ideology and Social Science*, London: Fontana.

Newfield, J. (1967) *The Prophetic Minority – the American New Left*, London: Anthony Blond.

Nicholls, G. (1898) *A History of the English Poor Law*, London: King and Son.

1991 Census (1993) *Ethnic Group and Country of Birth, Great Britain, Volume 2*, London: HMSO.

—— (1993) *County Report: Inner London (Part 2)*, London: HMSO.

Novak, T. (1988) *Poverty and the State: An Historical Sociology*, Milton Keynes: Open University Press.

O'Brien, M. and Penna, S. (1998) *Theorising Welfare*, London: Sage.

O'Connor, J. (1973) *The Fiscal Crisis of the State*, New York: St. Martin's Press.

Offe, C. (1984) *Contradictions of the Welfare State*, London: Hutchinson.

Oliver, J., Huxley, P., Bridges, K. and Mohamad, H. (1996) *Quality of Life and Mental Health Services*, London: Routledge.

Oliver, M. (1990) *The Politics of Disablement*, Basingstoke: Macmillan.

—— (1996) *Understanding Disability: From Theory to Practice*, Basingstoke: Macmillan.

Oliver, M. and Barnes, C. (1998) *Disabled People and Social Policy*, London: Longman.

Pacione, M. (1995) *Glasgow: The Socio-Spatial Development of the City*, Chichester: Wiley.

Palmer, B. D. (1990) 'The eclipse of materialism: Marxism and the writing of social history in the 1980's', in R. Miliband and L. Panitch (eds), *Socialist Register 1990: The Retreat of the Intellectuals*, London: Merlin Press.

Pelling, H. (1968) 'The working class and the origins of the welfare state' in H. Pelling, *Popular Politics and Society in Late Victorian Britain*, London: Macmillan.

Perkin, H. (1989) *The Rise of Professional Society: England Since 1880*, London: Routledge.

Perkins, R. (1997) 'Clubhouses – no thanks', *OpenMind* 88.

Petty, C., Roberts, D. and Smith, S. (1987) *Women's Liberation and Socialism*, London: Bookmarks.

Pierson, C. (1992) *Beyond the Welfare State*, Cambridge: Polity.

Pilgrim, D. (1990) 'Competing histories of madness', in R. Bentall (ed.), *Reconstructing Schizophrenia*, London: Routledge.

Pilgrim, D. and Rogers, A. (1993) *A Sociology of Mental Health and Illness*, Buckingham: Open University Press.

Pollack Petchesky, R. (1986) *Abortion and Women's Choice – the State, Sexuality and Reproductive Freedom*, London: Verso.

Ponting, C. (1994) *Churchill*, London: Sinclair Stevenson.

Poplar Council (1922) *Guilty and Proud of It: Poplar's Response*, London: Poplar Council.

Postgate, R. (1951) *The Life of George Lansbury*, London: Longmans, Green and Co.

Pound, J. (1971) *Poverty and Vagrancy in Tudor England*, London: Longman.

Power, A. and Tunstall, R. (1997) *Dangerous Disorder: Riots and Violent Disturbances in Thirteen Areas of Britain, 1991–92*, York: Joseph Rowntree Foundation.

Prashar, U. (1987) 'Too much talk and not enough positive action', in J. Benyon and J. Solomos (eds), *The Roots of Urban Unrest*, Oxford: Pergamon Press.

Profitt, R. (1984) 'Equal respect, equal treatment and equal opportunity', in J. Benyon (ed.), *Scarman and After*, Oxford: Pergamon Press.

Pugh, M. (1992) *Women and the Women's Movement in Britain 1914–1959*, Basingstoke: Macmillan.

Rae, J. (1890) 'State socialism and social reform', *Contemporary Review* 58: 435–54.

Ramdin, R. (1987) *The Making of the Black Working Class in Britain*, Aldershot: Gower.

Randall, V. (1987) *Women and Politics*, Basingstoke: Macmillan.

Rees, J. (1998) *The Algebra of Revolution*, London: Routledge.

Reicher, S. D. (1984) 'The St. Paul's riot: An explanation of the limits of crowd action in terms of a social identity model', *European Journal of Social Psychology* 14: 1–21.

—— (1996) ' "The battle of Westminster": Developing the social identity model of crowd behaviour in order to explain the initiation and development of collective conflict', *European Journal of Social Psychology* 26: 115–34.

Roberts, D. (1979) *Paternalism in Early Victorian England*, London: Croom Helm.

Robins, P. (1985) 'What is the government's employment policy?', *Economics* 21, Autumn: 113–15.

Rogers, A. (1988) 'Is there a new underclass?', *International Socialism* 40: 65–88.

Rogers, A. and Pilgrim, D. (1991) 'Pulling down churches: Accounting for the British mental health users' movement', *Sociology of Health and Illness* 13(2): 129–48.

—— (1996) *Mental Health Policy in Britain: A Critical Introduction*, Basingstoke: Macmillan.

Rogers, A., Pilgrim, D. and Lacey, R. (1993) *Experiencing Psychiatry: Users' Views of Services*, Basingstoke: Macmillan/MIND.

Rose, S. P. R., Lewontin, R. C. and Kamin. L. (1984) *Not in Our Genes*, Harmondsworth: Penguin.

Rosenberg, C. (1987) *1919 – Britain on the Brink of Revolution*, London: Bookmarks.

Ross, E. (1986) 'Labours of love: Rediscovering London working class mothers 1870–1914', in J. Lewis (ed.), *Labour and Love: Women's Experience of Home and Family*, Oxford: Blackwell.

Ross, L. (1998) 'African-American women and abortion', in R. Solinger (ed.), *Abortion Wars – A Half Century of Struggle*, California: University of California Press.

Rothstein, T. (1929) *From Chartism to Labourism*, London: Martin Lawrence.

Rowbotham, S. (1977) *Hidden from History – 300 Years of Women's Oppression and the Fight Against It*, London: Pluto Press.

Rowe, D. (1993) 'Foreword' to P. Breggin, *Toxic Psychiatry*, London: Harper Collins.

Rudé, G. (1964) *The Crowd in History 1730–1848*, London: Lawrence and Wishart.

Rule, J. B. (1988) *Theories of Civil Violence*, Berkeley: University of California Press.

Russell, D. (1977) *The Tamarisk Tree – My Quest for Liberty and Love, Volume 1*, London: Virago.

Russell, I. (1982) *Seventh Quarterly Report to Sir Robert McAlpine & Sons Ltd*, mimeo (private history of McAlpine's).

Ryan, P. (1978) ' "Poplarism" 1894–1930', in P. Thane (ed.), *The Origins of British Social Policy*, London: Croom Helm.

Saraga, E. (1998) (ed.) *Embodying the Social: Constructions of Difference*, London: Routledge/Open University.

Sassoon, M. and Lindow, V. (1995) 'Consulting and empowering black mental health service users', in S. Fernando (ed.), *Mental Health in a Multi-ethnic Society*, London: Routledge.

Saunders, P. (1981) *Social Theory and the Urban Question*, London: Hutchinson.

Saville, J. (1967) 'Unions and free labour: Background to Taff Vale decision', in A. Briggs and J. Saville (eds), *Essays in Labour History*, London: Macmillan.

—— (1983) 'The origins of the welfare state', in M. Loney, D. Boswell and J. Clarke (eds), *Social Policy and Social Welfare*, Milton Keynes: Open University Press.

Scarman, Lord (1981) *The Brixton Disorders: 10–12 April 1981*, Cmnd. 8427, London: HMSO.

Schneer, J. (1990) *George Lansbury*, Manchester: Manchester University Press.

Schulze-Gaevernitz, von, G. (1893) *Social Peace: A Study of the Trade Union in England*, London: Simpkin, Marshall, Hamilton and Kent.

Scottish Association for Mental Health (SAMH) (1998) *Attitudes to Mental Illness*, Edinburgh: SAMH.

Sedgewick, P. (1982) *Psychopolitics*, London: Pluto Press.

Segal, L. (1987) *Is the Future Female? Troubled Thoughts on Contemporary Feminism*, London: Virago.

Semmel, B. (1960) *Imperialism and Social Reform*, London: Allen and Unwin.

Shakespeare, T. (1993) 'Disabled people's self-organisation: A new social movement?', *Disability, Handicap and Society* 8(3): 249–64.

Sheldon, S. (1993) 'Who is the mother to make the judgement? The construction of women in English abortion laws', *Feminist Legal Studies* 1(1): 3–22.

Sheridan, T. with McAlpine, J. (1994) *A Time to Rage*, Edinburgh: Polygon.

Short, J. R. (1982) *Housing in Britain: The Post-War Experience*, London: Methuen.

Simms, M. (1992) 'Backstreet battles', *New Statesman and Society*, 23 October.

Sivanandan, A. (1981/2) 'From resistance to rebellion: Asian and Afro-Caribbean struggles in Britain', *Race and Class* XXIII(2/3): 111–52.

—— (1990) *Communities of Resistance*, London and New York: Verso.

Slack, P. (1988) *Poverty and Policy in Tudor and Stuart England*, London: Longman.

Smith, S. (1994) 'Mistaken identity – or can identity politics liberate the oppressed?', *International Socialism* 62: 3–50.

Solinger, R. (ed.) (1998) *Abortion Wars – A Half Century of Struggle 1950–2000*, California: University of California Press.

Solomos, J. (1986) 'Riots, urban protest and social policy: The interplay of reform and social control', *Policy Papers in Ethnic Relations*, no. 7, University of Warwick.

—— (1993) *Race and Racism in Britain*, Basingstoke: Macmillan.

Soper, K. (1990) *Troubled Pleasures. Writings on Politics, Gender and Hedonism*, London: Verso.

Stack, P. (1995) 'Equal access', *Socialist Review* 183: 14–15.

Stevenson, J. and Cook, C. (1977) *The Slump: Society and Politics During the Depression*, London: Quartet.

Stott, C. (1998) 'The inter-group dynamics of crowd events', in C. Barker and M. Tyldesley (eds), *Proceedings of the Fourth International Conference on Alternative Futures and Popular Protest*, April 1998, Manchester: MMU.

Strathclyde Anti-Poll Tax Federation (SAPTF) (1989) *The Coming of the Poll Tax*, Glasgow: SAPTF.

Sullivan, M. (1992) *The Politics of Social Policy*, London: Harvester Wheatsheaf.

—— (1996) *The Development of the British Welfare State*, Hemel Hempstead: Prentice Hall/Harvester Wheatsheaf.

Szasz, T. (1972) *The Myth of Mental Illness*, St Albans: Granada.

Tarrow, S. (1989) *Democracy and Disorder*, Oxford: Oxford University Press.

Taylor, S. (1984) 'The Scarman Report and explanation of riots', in J. Benyon (ed.), *Scarman and After*, Oxford: Pergamon Press.

Thane, P. (1982) 'The working class and state "welfare" in Britain, 1880–1914', *Historical Journal* 27(4): 877–900.

Thatcher, M. (1993) *The Downing Street Years*, London: Harper Collins.

Therborn, G. (1983) 'Why some classes are more successful than others', *New Left Review* 138: 37–55.

Thompson, E. P. (1963) *The Making of the English Working Class*, London: Victor Gollancz.

—— (1991) *Customs in Common*, London: Merlin Press.

Thompson, N. (1998) *Promoting Equality: Challenging Discrimination and Oppression in the Human Services*, Basingstoke: Macmillan.

Thompson, S. and Hoggett, P. (1996) 'Universalism, selectivism and particularism: Towards a post-modern social policy', *Critical Social Policy* 46: 21–43.

Timmins, N. (1996) *The Five Giants: A Biography of the Welfare State*, London: Fontana.

Tonge, J. (1995) 'Social movement or pressure group? The case of the poll tax', in C. Barker and M. Tyldsley (eds), *The Proceedings of the Conference on Alternative Futures and Popular Protest*, April 1995, Manchester: MMU.

Trades Union Congress (TUC) (1998) *Stress at Work*, October, TUC.

Trevelyan, G. M. (1972) *England in the Age of Wycliffe*, London: Longman.

Trotsky, L. D (1974 [1925]) 'Where is Britain going?', in R. Chappell and A. Clinton (eds), *Trotsky's Writings on Britain, Volume 2*, London: New Park.

Trotsky, L. D (1989) *On Black Nationalism and Self-Determination*, New York: Pathfinder Publications.

Vincent, D. (1991) *Poor Citizens. The State and the Poor in Twentieth Century Britain*, London: Longman.

Volosinov, V. (1986) *Marxism and the Philosophy of Language*, London: Harvard University Press.

Waddington, D. (1992) *Contemporary Issues in Public Disorder*, London and New York: Routledge.

Waddington, D., Jones, K. and Critcher, C. (1989) *Flashpoints: Studies in Public Disorder*, London and New York: Routledge.

Ward, C. (1991) *Influences: Voices of Creative Dissent*, Hartland Bideford, Devon: Green Books.

Warner, R. (1994) *Recovery from Schizophrenia: Psychiatry and Political Economy* (2nd edn.), London: Routledge.

Webb, S. (1890) 'The reform of the Poor Law', *Contemporary Review* 58: 95–120.

Westergaard, J. (1995) *Who Gets What?*, Cambridge: Polity.

Whiteside, N. (1991) *Bad Times*, London: Faber and Faber.

Wicks, H. (1992) *Keeping My Head: The Memoirs of a British Bolshevik*, London: Socialist Platform.

Willetts, D. (1992) *Modern Conservatism*, Harmondsworth: Penguin.

Williams, F. (1989) *Social Policy: A Critical Introduction*, Cambridge: Polity.

—— (1992) 'Somewhere over the rainbow: Universality and diversity in social policy', in N. Manning and R. Page (eds), *Social Policy Review 1991–92*, Canterbury: Social Policy Association.

—— (1996) 'Postmodernism, feminism and the question of difference', in N. Parton (ed.), *Social Theory, Social Change and Social Work*, London: Routledge.

Wilson, E. (1992) *A Very British Miracle*, London: Pluto Press.

Worsdall, F. (1979) *The Tenement: A Way of Life*, Edinburgh: W. and R. Chambers.

Wright, E. O. (1978) *Class, Crisis and the State*, London: Verso.

Young, J. D. (1989) *Socialism and the English Working Class. A History of English Labour 1883–1939*, London: Harvester.

Youngjohns, B. (1954) *Co-operation and the State*, Loughborough: Co-operative Union Education Department.

Name index

Subject index